Athletes at Risk: Drugs and Sport

Ray Tricker, Ph.D., and David L. Cook, Ph.D.

Funded in part by monies provided
by the Kansas Board of Regents
and the State of Kansas

 Wm. C. Brown Publishers

Copyright © 1990 by Wm. C. Brown Publishers. All rights reserved

Library of Congress Catalog Card Number: 89–60794

ISBN 0–697–10986–0

Printed in the United States of America by Wm. C. Brown Publishers,
2460 Kerper Boulevard, Dubuque, IA 52001

10 9 8 7 6 5 4 3 2 1

Contents

6. Dilemma of Drug Use for Maintenance and Rehabilitation, 93
James A. Hill, M.D.

7. Drug Abuse in College Athletics: The Role of Prevention and Intervention, 139
Ray Tricker, Ph.D.

List of Contributors

David L. Cook, Ph.D., is the Director of Sport Psychology at the University of Kansas.

Steven R. Heyman, Ph.D., is a professor in the Department of Psychology at the University of Wyoming.

James Hill, M.D., is an assistant professor of Orthopaedic Surgery at Northwestern University Medical School and Co-director of the center for Sports Medicine at Northwestern Memorial Hospital.

Rick McGuire, Ph.D., is the Head Track Coach and graduate professor of Sport Psychology in the Department of Health and Physical Education at the University of Missouri.

James Merdink, Pharm.D., is the Director of Drug Testing at American BioTech Laboratories.

Ray Tricker, Ph.D., is the Director of Drug Education in the Department of Health, Physical Education and Recreation at the University of Kansas.

Ralph A. Vernacchia, Ph.D., is an Associate Professor of Sport Psychology in the Department of Physical Education, Health, and Recreation at Western Washington University.

Bruce H. Woolley, Ph.D., is the Director of the Health Center at Brigham Young University.

James Wright, Ph.D., is President of Sports Science Consultants, Adirondack Life Group in Jay, New York.

Foreword

I am pleased to have the opportunity to comment on *Athletes at Risk: Drugs and Sport.* This much-needed book provides an indepth look at how our society's abuse of alcohol and other drugs impacts sports and athletes. Even more importantly, the authors present models for the prevention and reduction of drug abuse by athletes.

This book explores the special risks that athletes face and makes the following important points: (1) there is a significant drug problem in sports; (2) this problem parallels the drug abuse that has swept through society; (3) technological advances are creating ethical crises for players and coaches; (4) some athletes use drugs recreationally as well as to maintain fitness and to rehabilitate injuries; and (5) long term efforts to prevent, intervene and treat drug abuse are definitely needed. It details the roles of drug education, social skill enhancement, alternatives to drug use, drug-testing and sports psychology in combating drugs in sports.

I am very proud of the leadership in this area of University of Kansas professors Dr. Ray Tricker and Dr. David Cook, and of the Kansas Board of Regents, its staff, and member institutions. A scholarly work like *Athletes at Risk* is an excellent example of the commitment of our universities to a drug-free learning and sporting environment.

In the field of sports, alcohol and other drug abuse, addiction and alcoholism have wrecked far too many lives and destroyed too many careers. This book will help all who read it to understand what has created our dilemma and what must be done to prevent and reduce this national tragedy.

I am exceedingly proud that the state of Kansas and our comprehensive Toward A Drug-Free Kansas program have had a part in the development and publication of this book. On behalf of the citizens of Kansas I wish to express our sincere appreciation to the authors, contributors and to all who are working daily to make America drug-free.

Mike Hayden, Governor
State of Kansas

On March 26, 1987, Mike Hayden, Governor of Kansas, delivered a special message to the Kansas Legislature concerning drug and alcohol abuse. With specific reference to the public institutions of higher education governed and managed by the Kansas Board of Regents, the Governor discussed the state's obligation to its college students, their families and university supporters to assure them a drug-free learning environment at our state institutions.

He appointed a working Task Force chaired by Dr. David Waxman of the University of Kansas Medical Center; Regent Norman Jeter; Galen Davis, Special Assistant to the Governor on Substance Abuse Issues; Ted D. Ayres, General Counsel to the Board of Regents; and myself. He provided this specific charge to the Task Force:

"This group will focus on establishing consistent drug education, intervention, and support services to students at our Regents universities."

Numerous recommendations resulted from the efforts of the Task Force. With relation to intercollegiate athletics, one of the recommendations made to the Regents Institutions was:

"That athletic departments should continue to stress the educational aspects of their program for athletes."

Athletes at Risk: Drugs and Sport is a direct result of this recommendation.

Building upon research and enthusiasm provided by Professors Cook and Tricker, the Athletic Directors from our institutions with intercollegiate athletic programs, i.e., Emporia State University, Fort Hays State University, Kansas State University, Pittsburgh State University, the University of Kansas and Wichita State University, agreed to fund and support the publication of this book. This collective effort to provide an important educational resource for themselves, for Kansas and for the education community in general must be applauded. We believe the benefits from this effort will far exceed any individual campus effort which might have followed the charge of the Task Force.

Representatives from our institutions worked with Dr. Cook and Dr. Tricker to seek out individuals who were acknowledged as experts in their particular areas to serve as contributors to the book. It should also be noted that a commitment to the project and to the philosophy of the educational effort itself were factors equal in importance to scholarship and expertise. We are extremely pleased with the efforts of each individual author.

These are unsettling and worrisome times for intercollegiate athletics and, more importantly, for the student-athletes who currently participate, as well as those aspiring to do so in the future. While no one should doubt the benefits, both during college and after, of amateur athletic competition, many seem to have lost touch with the real spirit and purpose of competition; that they are, in fact, merely games.

It is hoped that *Athletes at Risk: Drugs and Sport* will assist in educating those who believe a competitive edge in athletics is justification for any action, no matter how dangerous. The Kansas Board of Regents is proud to be associated with this book and its publication. We are hopeful that it will serve to enlighten many future generations of student-athletes and educators.

Stanley Z. Koplik
Executive Director
Kansas Board of Regents

Preface

Drug abuse in sport has become a focus of concern for all who consider that the use of chemical substances as ergogenic aids is a serious threat to the well-being of athletes and the future of sporting competition. It is unfortunate that drug testing has also become a part of sport, but it appears that it is here to stay. For many athletes drug testing is considered an infringement of personal rights in which each individual is forced to prove innocence. However it is more unfortunate that most universities spend many thousands of dollars on drug testing while devoting little attention to drug education for their athletes. In fact, in a recent national survey, we observed that less than 5% of the NCAA division one universities provided more than two to three educational presentations per year about the use of drugs in sport. How unfortunate for the athlete!

Many athletes will compete for four years in a university athletic program without ever having the opportunity to examine the issues of drug use in sport in a well structured educational environment; with clear, unbiased information and careful guidance to develop healthy and safe decisions about drug use. It seems that most of the education received by athletes too often comes from drug marketeers and gymnasia where the bias is heavily in favor of use. In these settings athletes may feel encouraged to use chemical substances because of exaggerated and false promises. The poorly educated athlete may be more inclined to make uninformed and irrational decisions. As media reports have clearly indicated, unwise decisions can adversely affect the careers of athletes and in some cases jeopardize their lives.

It is important to educate athletes as comprehensively as possible about the drugs which are used in sport so that they can improve their ability to make responsible and healthy decisions; consequently these decisions must be based upon the best information we can provide. We can not realistically expect to legislate every decision an athlete makes in relation to drugs but hopefully we can help them develop a basis for saying: "No . . . I have a better way."

This text was developed with this purpose in mind. It is a product of several years of study related to the problems associated with drug abuse in sport and represents the thoughts of those who are professionally and personally concerned about this serious problem. Each chapter was written with a sincere commitment towards the health and well-being of athletes and a deep concern for the ramifications connected with drug abuse in sport.

This book follows closely the NCAA's recent commitment to education with the first extended drug education in sport program. This project culminated with a four-part video program and a workbook which was sent to every NCAA Athletic Department in the nation for the use of athletes and coaches. We were integrally involved in this NCAA Project as co-directors and we hope that this text also will complement the NCAA program and provide a further source of guidance and information. It is written specifically for coaches and athletes.

Today's coaches and athletes, who will influence the future generations of sport, need to take a stand in communicating to young athletes that they do not have to use drugs to succeed. Therefore we hope that the information provided in the following chapters will contribute to this stand as we attempt to promote a drug free future for sport where true athletic competition abounds, and an athlete's health and well-being is more important than "winning at all costs."

Ray Tricker   David L. Cook

Acknowledgments

We wish to offer special thanks to Ted Ayres, (General Counsel to the Kansas Board of Regents) for coordinating this project and enthusiastically supporting this text to its fruition.

We also wish to thank each of the Kansas Regents Institutions Athletic Directors for their commitment and financial support for this project. These included Bob Frederick: University of Kansas; Larry Travis (1987) and Steve Miller (1988): Kansas State University; Tom Shupe: Wichita State University; William Quayle: Emporia State University; Dennis Franchione: Pittsburg State University; and Robert Van Poppel: Fort Hays State University.

We also wish to thank members of the editorial review board which was established for this project. These included Carl Cramer: Athletic Trainer, Kansas State University; Marshall Havenhill: Director of Student Health, Emporia State University; Greg Buell: Coordinator of Clinical Counseling Services, Wichita State University; Al Ortolani: Athletic Trainer, Pittsburg State University; Richard Konzem: Assistant Athletic Director, University of Kansas; and Lynn Bott: Athletic Trainer, University of Kansas.

Finally we would like to express our appreciation to Wayne Osness: Chairman of the Dept. of HPER, here at Kansas University for encouraging us to pursue this opportunity and for providing the resources needed to complete this project.

CHAPTER 1

ATHLETES AT RISK

Rick McGuire, Ph.D.

Stories of drug use and abuse are commonplace in sports today. Drugs which have been used both in an attempt to enhance athletic performance as well as those used for more recreational purposes continue to command widespread national media attention. Collegiate athletes being disqualified from major football bowl games, NFL and NBA players being suspended from play in their respective leagues, and even the dramatic deaths of prominent college and professional athletes—all drug related incidents—have become commonplace headlines on our sports pages. Even the recent Olympic Games in Seoul, Korea, with the disqualification of several gold medalists for their use of banned drugs, riveted the attention of sports enthusiasts world-wide to the realization that widespread substance abuse does exist in sport. While some still respond with shocked disbelief, all indications are that we have presently only uncovered the "tip of a very large iceberg."

This issue of drugs in sport poses extremely important and urgent questions which must be addressed by those who are involved in athletics. It is recognized that with the incredible focus of media attention and the public's near fixation on athletics, there exists the possibility that the degree of the problem may be distorted or blown out of proportion. Yet at the same time, those who are experienced in and knowledgeable of athletics, of athletes and their behaviors, and of the athletic environment, would be naive if they could not recognize and admit that there is a very real issue.

As this text attempts to provide the most current information and understanding regarding the wide range of issues in drug abuse and athletics, it will be the intent of this first chapter to focus directly on the athlete. What is it about our athletes, and the athletic environment, that causes them to be a population at risk in regards to drug usage? Three distinct categories of issues will be addressed in the attempt to develop a sensible understanding and answer for such a complex question. These categories include: (1) issues related to athletic performance, (2) issues related to the *person* of the athlete, and (3) issues related to the athletic leadership that provides the athletic experience for our athletes.

Drugs: Are They Really a Problem in Sport?

Yes!

No more should ever need to be said. But we are a society which demands evidence, and such evidence is difficult to obtain on this issue. Several studies of the incidence of drug usage amongst athletes have reported wide ranges in the percentages of users, anywhere from 2% to over 20% (Tricker and Cook 1988; Heitzinger et al. 1986; Anderson and McKeag 1985). At the same time, results of drug testing conducted by several organizations, such as the NCAA, the USOC, individual collegiate institutions, and several sport governing bodies, tend to confound the issue even further, as they often generate results which raise more questions than they answer.

Yes! Drugs really are a problem in sport! In fact, they are a problem in life in general. They permeate all aspects of our society. From the industrial shop to the executive suite, an estimated one out of six people in the work force abuse drugs (Manning 1988). If sport really is a reflection of life, then drugs are a problem in sport.

But the biggest and most resounding YES of all comes from the athletes themselves. They know that drugs are a problem in sport. They know that they compete against other athletes who are, or have been, involved with drug usage. They know that they also face the often difficult question of whether or not to use drugs themselves. From football to track and field, from swimming to weight lifting, from basketball to power lifting, from biking to baseball, from soccer to shooting, athletes from the international level, professional level, collegiate level and, even most alarmingly of all, athletes at the high school level are using and abusing drugs (Strauss 1988).

Yes! Drugs are really a problem in sport!

Why Do Athletes Use Drugs?

This is a highly complex question, and there is obviously no simple, complete, and easily generalized answer. People who are not athletes, just people in general, use drugs for many reasons. Just a few of these reasons may include: to cope with threats to self-esteem, resulting in such emotions as anger, frustration, or fear; because of the novelty or for the fun; to gain some sort of an edge; as a result of peer pressures; or sometimes even just because "they are there."

Athletes are people, too. Thus, all of these reasons may, and do, fit athletes as well. But athletes are a special people, living and participating in a highly charged and intense environment. What might it be about this environment, or about the personal qualities of the athletes, that may contribute to their being a population at risk of abusing drugs?

Performance Enhancement: The Affects and the Effects

Issues related to athletic performance enhancement focus on the *affects* and the *effects* of drug usage in sport. There obviously is an incredible desire, and even demand, for creating and generating the greatest optimal performance on the part of athletes. This demand may cause many to turn to any means available which might bring the desired increase in capability and satisfy the compulsion to achieve optimal performance.

Unfortunately, this has caused some athletes to go beyond the more accepted and appropriate avenues of achieving, such as scientifically sound training and conditioning programs, the use of the most modern state-of-the-art equipment, the development of better sport skills and techniques, or the more effective use of the mind and highly refined mental skills. Instead, they may turn to more of a quick-fix approach; that is, turning to the use of chemicals or other substances that could possibly generate a greater increased capability in a much shorter period of time.

Athletes who choose the route of substance supplementations such as anabolic steroids with their training, believe that there will be two main benefits derived: (1) the stimulation of actual tissue growth to achieve greater muscle size and strength, and (2) the facilitation of recovery time following intense training sessions, thus allowing for more frequent training sessions with more intense training loads.

Some experts question the validity of these benefits. But this is not the question nor the issue. The reality is that the athletes, either rightfully

3

or wrongfully, do perceive that such benefits are available through the use of these substances. In their desire to do "whatever it takes" to achieve these training affects, to meet the necessary athletic performance demands, to attain the athletic achievement of their own dreams, and to satisfy the demands of their public, many athletes are tempted, and all too many turn, to the use of such substances!

It is estimated that over one million athletes today are taking drugs such as anabolic steroids (Duda 1986). Some reports from former NFL athletes imply the staggering figure that upwards of 75% of those athletes use steroids (Johnson 1985).

While in the past it was common knowledge that many athletes were taking steroids, not many in the sports world gave much consideration to the problems of steroid usage. Only recently have sport regulatory organizations begun to take serious action to address the issue of steroids in sport. According to John Toner, Chairman of the NCAA's Drug Testing Committee, "steroids are probably our most serious problem in intercollegiate athletics today" (University of Minnesota 1988). An even more alarming trend is the downward spread to younger age groups of drug usage to improve performance. All indications are that the use of steroids by high school athletes is on the rise (Strauss 1988).

Along with the use of drugs to affect an enhanced performance, athletes also turn to drug usage to help them to deal and cope with the effects of their athletic training and competitions. This may cause the use of substances to aid in the rehabilitation and recovery from pains, strains, sores, injuries, and possibly even from the psychological and mental fatigue that often accompanies sport participation. Dealing with these effects of sport may allow athletes to return to training or competing the next day more confident in their ability to meet their new challenges and demands. Drugs may provide a shortcut in this process and, along with it, a deluded or clouded sense of personal well-being and confidence.

But for issues related to the affects and effects of performance enhancement, it is also quite evident that athletes involve themselves in the use of a variety of substances in an attempt to generate a greater performance capability and to deal with the effects of their training and performance load.

Recreational Uses: Environmental Exposures

Successful athletes live in an athletic environment which is rather unique relative to that of the nonathletic population. This environment offers exposures for these athletes which could very well contribute to the influence to use drugs. The eye of public scrutiny, the media attention, the incredible societal focus on sport generally, and certainly on the revenue producing and entertainment oriented sports, particularly football and basketball, leave athletes experiencing a *fish bowl* effect. Most other individuals never have the opportunity to experience anything like this with any regularity, and certainly not with the emotional intensity as do athletes. Every play, every action, every behavior, and every emotion are everybody's business and are open for public scrutiny and critical evaluation. When all goes well, life can be wonderfully exciting and rewarding for the athlete. But when things come up short of the public's expectations, it could seem like the world is incredibly unfair and that there is nowhere to hide.

Along with this public exposure and the almost bigger than life effects it has for athletes, often comes the availability for new social opportunities. Spectators and sports fans put athletes upon a pedestal. Athletes are special people, and as special people they are provided with a variety of new social opportunities and social contacts. They are invited to functions, to parties, to social events, and at these events they may find many new *friends*. These friends may be quick to provide the opportunity for the availability and use of alcohol, marijuana, cocaine, and other socially related *goodies*. These new friends bring new peer pressures, new temptations. With their normal desires to be accepted and gain the benefits of belonging, the athletes' decision-making processes may become clouded. Drug usage may soon follow for many.

The Athlete as a Person

Self-esteem

Many psychologists and drug and alcohol counselors believe that individuals involve themselves in substance abuse because they lack a good strong positive sense of self-esteem. It is important for all of us to have positive self-esteem, that is, to feel good about ourselves, and to feel a sense of self-worth.

While to describe all that goes into an individual's development and evaluation of their self-worth would be extremely complex, it can be reduced to a few simple concepts with which most individuals can relate with an immediate and strong personal identification. Essentially, in-

5

dividuals gain a sense of self-worth, of being worthy, as three fundamental needs are fulfilled. These needs are:

1. The need to feel *competent,*
2. The need to feel *achieving,*
3. The need to feel *accepted* or *loved.*

For most individuals the ability to perform an important task with the required or desired level of competence, whether it be a skill in the workplace, home, or hobby, brings with it a good sense of self-worth. People feel good about themselves when they can demonstrate and be recognized by others as being competent. This feeling of self-worth is enhanced as the competence leads to notable achievement, often with some direct relationship between higher levels of achievement and even greater feelings of self-esteem. This sense of self-worth becomes complete, even validated, when this competence and achievement brings with it the love, respect, and acceptance of important others. This lets individuals feel like they are *good* and that they really *fit.*

Sport provides a tremendously fertile set of opportunities for its participants to gain great senses of self-worth. First of all, with the tremendous priority in our society places on being an athlete, there are greater and more readily available payoffs for the athlete than possibly in any other segment of society. Secondly, sport is all about developing and demonstrating skills, that is, proving one's level of competence. These skills are usually very identifiable, and athletes are able to recognize improvements in skill levels and feel great about themselves as they attain new levels.

Athletes then use these skills, either individually or in concert with a team, in some form of competition leading to the chance for achievement. This achievement, of course, is usually measured in the form of *winning.* Athletes are conditioned to feel great when they win. Much of this reinforcement comes from the public, which follows their competitions with great interest and intensity. The ultimate achievement is to be the final winner, the champion, the winningest winner of them all. To this athlete or team comes great public prominence, with the individuals involved experiencing a tremendous sense of competence, achievement, love, and acceptance. Thus, they have gained from sport a great feeling of self-worth!

Eventually, however, athletes and other sport participants find that sport and its public are extremely *fickle lovers.* While in a given moment sport can provide the affirmation of great self-esteem, it can all become shattered very quickly.

For example, one of the achievements and honors gained by star athletes at any level of competition is the opportunity to move up to the next level, whether such a move is from the junior varsity to the varsity, from high school to college, or from college to the professional ranks. Such opportunities come about most often because the athletes have been extremely competent and have demonstrated great achievements at their previous levels.

At the new level, however, they often find that everybody has their same skill level or, in many cases, are even more skilled. While they previously enjoyed displaying their competence and producing great achievements, they now may find that they lack confidence, aren't quite as talented as they'd like to be, and may find themselves dealing with failure and frustration much more regularly than achievement. They now may also sense that their coaches and teammates do not feel confident in their ability, and feel a bit on the outside of things. This can be difficult, even embarrassing, especially when the public no longer has the opportunity to share its adulation, or worse, looks upon these athletes with scorn or ridicule as if they were *losers.*

While this scenario may seem a bit extreme at first, it should also be recognized as being the typical experience of many athletes. In fact, our most talented athletes are almost certainly destined to experience this side of sport as they have greater opportunities to move up to higher levels of competition.

Athletes invest such an enormous amount of time, energy, and emotion into their sport effort that much of their personal identity is tied up in and defined by their sport performances and achievements.

Coupled with the tremendous intensities of sport competition and the public's emotional involvement, athletes can and do experience extreme swings in their own sense of self-esteem and self-worth. The resulting emotional instability, an unfortunate natural outcome of intense sport involvement, leaves athletes vulnerable to the temptation to cope through the use of drugs.

Risk Takers and Thrill Seekers

At risk of potentially overgeneralizing a bit, it is very important to acknowledge that high-level competitive athletes may very well have some characteristics in their personalities that make them quite different from those in the normally, nonathletic population. This is often difficult for the public to understand and accept. When it comes to the athletic field, the public does not want its athletes to display *normal* behaviors at all. In fact, it expects absolutely *abnormal* behaviors, desiring its athletes to be nothing short of spectacular. In statistical terminology, great athletes would display behaviors and characteristics that would place them nearly off the normal curve—at the third or fourth standard deviation above the mean—or further.

To be great athletes takes individuals with a willingness to commit themselves to incredible numbers of hours, weeks, months, years, and in some cases even decades, to their sport involvement and development. This investment often comes with little or no probability of significant financial reward, and in many cases requires an enormous financial expense. To become great athletes, it requires individuals who are willing to ride the emotional roller coaster of extreme highs and devastating lows, and to regularly place themselves and their egos on the competitive firing line, exposing themselves not only to the athletic challenges from their opponents but to the critical eye of public scrutiny as well.

Yes, it certainly takes some very special individuals to stand the heat in the crucible of athletic competition. These individuals are the epitome of what could be described as *thrill seekers* and *risk takers*. They are possibly filled with and driven by a near *delusion of invulnerability*. Great athletes, athletes who consistently achieve a the highest levels, the champions of whom legends are made, possess abnormal levels of these types of characteristics. That is part of what allows them to be great. And the public loves them for it!

Yet that same public, as well as the athletes themselves, are often naively frustrated and uncomfortable when these same athletes act and behave abnormally outside of sport in the real world. These same high levels of such characteristics as thrill seeking, risk taking, and the delusion of one's own invulnerability are what drive these individuals to behave in ways different from most people and to involve themselves in activities that are not always in the normally accepted mainstream.

Similarly, it is these same characteristics, these bigger than life perceptions that are intensely reinforced by an adoring athletic public, that leave our athletes acutely vulnerable to the temptations of becoming involved with drugs. To experience in yet another way the intense highs, to gain a new thrill, to take the chance of living on the edge—always confident that the tragic consequences will once again be escaped—this is the essence of life for many athletes. Unfortunately, all are not so lucky.

8

The Post Patterns

Many athletes, maybe even most athletes, are able to effectively cope with themselves and with life as long as they are intensely involved with their sport activity. There are at least three critical periods when this active involvement ceases and the athletes' vulnerability for involvement in drug usage increases. These periods can be referred to as the athletes' *post patterns,* alluding to the athletes' post-game, post-season, and post-career activities.

For many sports and in many towns and settings, the post-game party is almost as much a part of sport as the game itself. To quote a hit tune from a previous era, many athletes (as well as coaches, parents, and fans) believe that "... You can't have one without the other!" Partying after the game, either in joyous celebration of victory or for the commiseration and consolation after defeat, is an often accepted and even religiously reinforced tradition. In decades and generations of the past, beer may have been the accepted beverage or drug of choice. Times have changed, and it is quite possible these drugs of choice may have changed as well. But it is quite safe to say that athletes still find their way to post-game parties.

The post-season offers a difficult challenge for some athletes. During the season, their lives are neatly scheduled and disciplined. They are busy in activities in which they find both identification and enjoyment and the opportunity to expend tremendous amounts of physical and emotional energies. After the season, though, there is often a void which some find difficult to fill with positive involvements and appropriate activities. These unfilled idle hours may leave athletes vulnerable to the alluring invitation to indulge in drugs.

Facing their post-career life is a difficult challenge for many outstanding athletes. Having spent an enormous percentage of their lives training for and competing in athletics, many athletes have neglected to prepare themselves for a meaningful professional career upon their retirement. Not only are they possibly lacking the education or skills to make their place in the work world, they often miss the intensity of emotional charge and ego reward their sport careers had provided. So much of their egos and identities were defined by their athletic prowess and the camaraderie of their teammates and competitors, that nothing in the real world can quench their thirst for more. Some literally drift through a hollow and empty life, still searching for their next big game and championship ring, always reliving the past, and failing to grow and move on into a productive and fulfilling post-career life. This same scenario is even more traumatic when an athlete's career has been terminated unexpectedly and prematurely due to injury.

These individuals, lacking preparation and counseling for life after sport, face a potentially enormous identity crisis, a serious threat to their perceived self-esteem, and may find themselves extremely vulnerable to becoming seriously involved with drugs.

The Role of Athletic Leadership

To this point, the discussion of drugs and sport in regards to athletes as a population at risk has focused on developing descriptions and understandings of the athletes as individuals, their motivations for behavior, and the demands of the athletic environment. Attention will now be turned to an extremely important, yet often over-looked or under estimated, factor contributing to athletes being at risk for involvement with drugs. This factor is isolated in the role of the athletic leadership, in the individuals who provide the leadership in defining and determining the quality of the sport experiences that athletes receive.

Who are these athletic leaders? For sure, they include the coaches. Athletics and athletes meet at the coach. So much of the quality of the experiences that athletes receive is determined by the quality of the leadership of the coaches who provide those experiences. Along with coaches, the athletic leaders in question here may also include the athletic trainers and even the athletic directors. More specifically, attention is pointed to athletic leaders who fit into the following categories:

1. Leaders who *instruct* drug usage,
2. Leaders who *allow* drug usage,
3. Leaders who *cover* drug usage,
4. Leaders who are the *providers of the caines.*

Leaders Who Instruct Drug Usage

This may come as a shock to many, but if we are to get serious about the issue of drugs in sport, we must be willing to admit that there are many coaches who are directly instructing their athletes in the use of drugs. The instruction is primarily in the use of anabolic steroids or other strength, growth, or training enhancing substances. In some cases the coaches directly provide these drugs to their athletes. Few people in the athletic environment have greater direct influence on the values and be-

10

haviors of athletes than do their coaches. Without question, these athletic leaders place their athletes directly at risk.

Leaders Who Allow Drug Usage

Although even a few is still too many, certainly the number of coaches or athletic leaders who are directly instructing the use of anabolic steroids or other such substances in sport is relatively small. However, there is a much larger number of sport leaders who, while not directly instructing drug usage, may be aware of, or suspect its use, and turn their heads the other way allowing such usage to continue while failing to provide counsel for the athletes who are involved.

Compelled by their need for their athletes to develop and maintain competitiveness with the opposition, coaches praise, reward, and reinforce athletes for tremendous gains in size or strength, failing to follow through on their own suspicions that these growths were enhanced by illegal substances. Wherever this is allowed, the coaches' action, or lack of action, is affirmation that whatever it takes—even if it means drugs—is allowable. Athletes wishing to remain competitive get the message loud and clear. Unwittingly, they find themselves facing a decision as members of a population very much at risk.

Leaders Who Cover Drug Usage

Athletes are very much a population placed at risk by the leaders in sport who have provided evidence that hides the truth about athlete involvement in drug use. In the past few years the drug testing of athletes, especially in the NCAA collegiate programs and at international athletic events, has become quite standard. It would appear that these drug testing programs have arisen out of some strong suspicions and evidences that the participating athletes were, indeed, involved with drugs. While the initial intent of such programs was to inhibit the use of illegal anabolic steroids and other such performance enhancing substances, costs of such in many cases have proven to be prohibitive. Current testing has focused more directly on the use of marijuana, cocaine, amphetamines, and others.

Typically, the reports of these drug testing programs, especially those from the collegiate institutions, have uncovered only an incredibly small percentage of users, often 2% or less. This is in marked contrast to the more generally accepted figures for college campuses and college-aged populations ranging anywhere from 20% to 40%, or even higher.

If, in fact, less than 2% of our athletic population is involved in drug usage as compared to the much higher percentages for the regular population, then a logical conclusion may be that athletics is a great intervention for eliminating or reducing substance abuse on the part of individuals. But if, in fact, these figures are inaccurate; and if, in fact, the incidence of drug usage is much higher than the 2%, then these figures are dangerously distorting and covering the severity of the issue.

Those involved with young people in athletics on a regular basis are quite confident that there is a higher percentage of participation in substance abuse than the reported 2%. Thus, the leaders who continue to generate and provide documentation of that ridiculously low percentage are, in fact, covering the issue and diverting our attention from really addressing the issue of drugs in sport. This must change if sport leaders are ever to involve themselves in realistically serving to remediate the drug related problems within our athletic population.

The leaders who cover the issue of drug usage in sport, for whatever reasons or in whatever ways, serve only to increase the risk for all of the athletic participants.

Leaders Who Are the Providers of the Caines

The fourth and final focus on the role of athletic leadership points to those leaders who are the providers of the *caines*. Of course these are not the candy canes, because they are not candy at all. Instead, these "caines" include such items as Novocaine, Procaine, and any of the other similar substances used to deaden the athlete's physical pains on a Friday night or a Saturday afternoon when it is determined that it is so important that the athlete play. In such settings, athletes learn quickly that, in spite of injury, the need to win is so great that an injection of a drug to deaden the pain is acceptable.

Even if such pain killers were provided as good, safe, and ethical medical practice, as one would hope and assume that they are, there still remains a very confusing mixed message for the athlete. If it is acceptable, even encouraged, that athletes use a "caine" during the day to deaden a pain in their leg and to accept that it is right to do so, then why would we expect that athletes should conclude that it is wrong for them to use another "caine"—Cocaine—in the evening to deaden another pain they are experiencing in their heads or in their hearts?

12

The leaders who provide the "caines" are, in fact, placing our athletes at risk. In some unfortunate cases they are at possible risk for further injury or debilitation as a result of the masking of a physical pain in a performance setting. Most certainly they are at risk in the question of substance use and abuse in general.

Unfortunately, we must be willing to admit that there are coaches and leaders in the world of sport today who, for whatever reasons—a compelling need to produce winners, to save their jobs, to generate greater revenues, or some other situationally specific factors—are directly contributing to their athletes being at risk for involvement with drug abuse.

The Role of the Public

In each and every aspect of the analyses provided, the role of the public, in placing the athletes at risk in regards to the use and abuse of drugs, has been either directly stated, strongly alluded to, or inherently implied. Our society is obsessed with sport and with athletes. More accurately stated: society is obsessed with winning in sport and with winning athletes.

The tangible and intangible rewards provided for those who attain such distinction are great, but the price that many pay is often devastating. Again, the recent Olympic Games in Seoul provide us with too many disturbing examples of where being an Olympian was not enough, or where even winning the silver or bronze medals was considered to be failure. Being the very best, bringing home the gold, and becoming the ultimate winner were all that mattered. The payoff is for the one who wins! Yes, the public certainly plays an important role in placing athletes in a position of risk.

This is not to relieve the athletes of their own personal decision making responsibilities. Athletes comprise a very special group of individuals, with a very special and intensely challenging set of demands. At the same time, they also receive many very special opportunities and rewards. From those to whom much is given, much is also required.

Summary

Yes, our athletes are a population at risk. Yes, our athletes are using and abusing drugs and other such substances. These are very real issues and require intensive study to build better and deeper understandings. Genuine answers will not be developed by studying athletes alone, but by also focusing on key issues related to providing positive and effective athletic leadership through coaches and others. There will be no quick fix answer for issues related to drugs and sport. Our hopes for the future rest in the provision of comprehensive educational programs delivered through competent, caring and committed sport leaders.

References

Anderson, W. A. and McKeag, D. B. (1985) *The substance use and abuse habits of college athletes.* Michigan State University College of Human Medicine. A paper presented to NCAA Athletic Council Executive Comittee, Drug Education Committee.

Chappell, J.N. (1987) *Drug use, and abuse in the athlete.* In *Sport psychology: The psychological health of the athlete,* ed. J.R. May and M.J. Asken. New York: PMA Publishing Corp.

Duda, M. (1986) Do anabolic steroids pose an ethical dilemma for US physicians? (Should they prescribe and monitor?) *Physician and Sportsmedicine* 14.

Heitzinger, et al. (1986) *Data collection and analysis high school, college, professional athletes alcohol/drug survey.* Heitzinger and Associates, 333 W. Miflin, Madison, WI 53703.

Johnson, W.D. (1985) Steroids: A problem of huge dimensions. *Sports Illustrated* 62.

Manning, S. (1988) Drugs: A national crisis. *Scholastic Update* 120.

University of Minnesota Department of Intercollegiate Athletics. (1988) *Steroids are big trouble: An anti-steroid abuse campaign.* Unpublished Manuscript. Minneapolis.

Reedy, G. (1982) Drug abuse in sports: Denial fuels the problem. *Physician and Sportsmedicine* 10(4):114–123.

Strauss, R.H. (1988) Drug abuse in sports: A three pronged response. *Physician and Sportsmedicine* 16(2):47.

Tricker, R. and Cook, D. (1988) The current status of drug intervention in college athletic programs. *Journal of Alcohol and Drug Education.* In press.

CHAPTER 2

HISTORY AND EVOLUTION OF DRUGS IN SPORT

Bruce H. Woolley, Ph.D.

Historical Overview

Drug taking to increase an athlete's chance of winning has reached pandemic proportions. Drug use has been documented in all sports which require speed, strength, size, endurance, and concentration. Once an athlete performs well after taking a particular substance, he/she will give the credit for the enhanced result to the drug. Others are then told about this perceived result from the drug and many begin taking it. At that point the practice becomes almost impossible to stop unless numerous deaths are directly attributed to the ingestion of the substance.

Modern athletes use a greater variety of drugs than ever before. In a survey of drug use by athletes in Florida, it was noted that athletes were "eager to try any drug or substance promoted by anyone claiming improved performance by use of the substance." Moreover, the athletes obtained these medications from drug wholesalers, drug representatives, pharmacists, veterinarians, other athletes, and illicit blackmarket sources, only rarely consulting a physician for a prescription (Taylor 1984).

The growth of drug use in sports has paralled the changes that have swept society. Cocaine and anabolic steroids were at one time used only by elite amateur and professional athletes. Now there are reports that cocaine is the drug of choice among eighteen to twenty-five-year old athletes and nonathletes, and that anabolic steroid use is increasing in prepubertal males and in male and female athletes from high school age and up. It has been estimated that one of every eight athletes in the United States may have a current or potentially significant problem with drug dependence (Donovan 1983).

15

As drug use and abuse continues, it is apparent that sex-biased differences in drug use among athletes are rapidly vanishing. Kit Saunders, director of women's sports for the University of Wisconsin, speaking at the University's First National Training Institute on Sports, Alcohol, and Drug Abuse, predicted that "drug use by women will follow the same pattern that it has for men." During her presentation, she related the statistics that nearly one in four of Big Ten coaches have reported excessive social use of alcohol by their teams, and that fourteen percent of high school coaches have reported helping their female athletes seek professional help for drinking problems (Reedy 1982).

Many people have expressed that drug use to achieve greater athletic achievement is a new phenomenon and that we should revert back to the good old days, but that is a simplistic outlook. The use of substances for performance enhancement has existed since the dawn of man's history. Even the most primitive people developed potions that could induce changes in their bodies and thoughts. In fact, almost all cultures have evidenced a desire, whether conscious or unconscious, to flee from monotony, frustration, and pain, and to seek euphoria. However, despite the vast variety of intoxicating properties that these early substances possessed, the predominant use was to produce a mystical or communal experience with various perceived deities. Undoubtedly, some of the substances were also used for medicinal purposes and physiological enhancement.

The ingenuity that people possess to discover natural or synthetic substances that can alter consciousness and enhance physiological performance levels seems to be inexhaustible. Even substances used anciently are still advocated to athletes as being effective in the pursuit of greater athletic achievement. Much has been passed down through legendary lore.

Anemones, which according to Greek myth sprang from the blood of Adonis after he was mortally wounded by a boar, were used to cure colds, gout, leprosy, and to lengthen longevity. Betony, named after Beronice, a woman healed by Christ, was believed to cure almost all ills of the body and the soul, to enhance sexual prowess, and as an aid to reduce recovery time after exertion. Blackberry brambles were legendarily used by Christ to drive out the money changers from the temple, and children were at one time passed through a bramble arch as a cure for rickets and to help them be fleet of foot. Bryony, used by witches in spells, was taken as a purgative and is still considered a potent aphrodisiac.

When God caused a deep sleep to fall on Adam to remove a rib from which Eve would be created, the Old Testament indicates that this was accomplished by using mandrake. The mandrake root, like its relatives in the Solanaceae family (deadly nightshade, jimpson weed, henbane), contains a number of atropine-like alkaloids. The mandrake has been used as a sedative, a hypnotic, an analgesic during surgery, or as an aphrodisiac. Athletes have used it in an effort to restart the body's testosterone production after anabolic steroid use.

Eyebright, which was thought to have been rubbed on Adam's eyes to permit him to see the future mortality of man, is still used by modern herbalists and athletic trainers for eye complaints. In popular tradition viper's bugloss was believed to help lumbago, relieve aches and pains from excess activity, and increase milk production in nursing mothers. The ancient Egyptians felt that runners could continue the pace much further if they ingested ground-up rear hooves of the Abyssinian ass that had been flavored with rose hips. However, only during the last century have we started to know something about the pharmacology and chemistry of some of these substances and their effects on performance (Woolley 1983).

The ancient Olympics were started by the Greeks in 776 B.C., and the winner of each race would have a wreath of laurel placed on his head. The ancient Greeks believed that sport was a religious, moral, and civic undertaking. Sport, they said, is morally serious because a noble aim of life is the appreciation of worthy things, such as beauty and bravery. These games were carried out for about 1000 years until they were discontinued by the Romans. The Romans felt that the athletes were becoming too professional and that substances were being used in an effort to enhance performance. This, the Romans felt, devalued the true meaning and value of athletic competition. The employment of various drugs to enhance physical and mental capabilities in Olympic competition had been reported as early as the third century B.C., when some Greek athletes were said to have used mushrooms and animal protein (meat) to improve their performance in competition (Hanley 1979).

By the 19th century, many substances had been used by athletes in hopes of improving their performance and obtaining an advantage over their competition. Cactus-based stimulants, caffeine, ether-dipped sugar cubes, nitroglycerin, opium, and doctors who followed marathoners on bicycles to administer brandy laced with strychnine are some examples of such substances (Donovan, 1983)

17

International Federations and Olympic Problems

The awareness of drug use in the modern Olympics probably began during the 1904 games in St. Louis. It took four physicians to revive Tom Hanks after he won the marathon. It was later discovered that he had taken a large dose of strychnine and brandy just before he began the race (Goldman 1984).

During the 1952 Winter Games in Oslo, Olympic officials found numerous syringes and broken ampules in the locker room of the speed skaters. The ampules had contained amphetamines and engendered significant controversy. However, no concerted action was taken to prevent or stop this type of *cheating* until years later.

On the opening day of the 1960 Games in Rome, a Danish cyclist, Knud Jensen, collapsed during team trials and died. It was later revealed that he had been taking nicotinyl alcohol in combination with amphetamines. Dick Howard, a 400-meter hurdler, died at the same games from heroin overdose and toxicity.

At the commencement of the 1964 Games in Tokyo, it was observed that the body structure of some of the Eastern bloc athletes was significantly more muscular than at previous competitions. These athletes were also up to 1 1/2 inches taller. It was suspected that these athletes were using anabolic steroids and various other drugs to achieve this physiological advantage.

In response to this rise of drug use and the drug-related demise of several Olympic athletes, the First European Drug Colloquium was held in Uriage, Belgium, in the fall of 1965. Out of this meeting a resolution was written and presented to the International Olympics Committee. The adoption of this resolution, called the IOC Regulation 27, defined drug doping, established a medical commission, created a list of banned drugs, and outlined a rough procedure for testing athletes for the presence of any of these drugs in their urine. Drug doping was defined as,

> the administration of or use by a competing athlete of any substance foreign to the body, or any physiological substance taken in abnormal quantity or taken by an abnormal route of entry into the body with the sole intention of increasing in an artificial and unfair manner his/her performance in competition. When necessity demands medical treatment with any substance which because of its nature, dosage, or application is able to boost the athlete's performance in competition in an artificial and unfair manner, this too is regarded by the IOC as doping (USOC Sportsmediscope).

Further regulation became possible during this same year (1965), as Beckett first applied sensitive gas chromatographic testing procedures to control drug abuse at an athletic event (Catlin 1987).

By the 1968 Olympics in Mexico City, the use of drugs to enhance athletic performance had become a serious problem internationally and drug testing was instituted for the first time. F. Don Miller, then the executive director of the United States Olympic Committee, in announcing the strict drug testing program, stated:

> This is the first step in our war against the use of drugs by our athletes, but not a war against our fine young men and women. We must wipe out this danger once and for all and obliterate the image of the 'chemical athlete' that is starting to shape itself in the public mind.

At the 1972 Olympic games in Munich, the female swimmers from the United States outclassed the world. These athletes won eight gold medals, five silver, and four bronze. The East German swimmers won four silver and two bronze. The following year the First World Swimming Championships were held in Belgrade, Yugoslavia. The teams were basically the same people as those who had participated in the Munich Games the preceding year. However, the East German swimmers had gained an average of twenty-two pounds of lean body mass and were, on the average, 1 1/2 inches taller. The U.S. women swimmers won only three gold medals, while the East German women won ten of the possible fourteen gold medals and set seven world records. The 1972 Olympics also provided the first disqualification and loss of a medal by an American. A sixteen-year-old male swimmer from the U.S., Rick De-Mott, was disqualified and lost his gold medal because he tested positive for an anti-asthmatic drug which had been prescribed for him by his physician.

Just prior to the 1976 Olympic games in Montreal, the IOC presented an extensive manual of banned substances (Percy 1978). In the pre-Olympic camp, nine of twenty-four swimmers tested positive for banned substances. Seven of the twenty-four were from the United States. However, the level of sophistication in the laboratory did not match that of the athlete using the drugs, and few athletes who used drugs from the banned list were caught during the actual games. Moreover, there were inconsistencies among the national and international sport governing bodies as to how and when testing would occur and what, if any, penalties would be enforced (Connolly 1984).

19

The United States did not participate in the 1980 games held in Moscow. However, drug testing was conducted utilizing radioimmunoassay procedures that employ enzyme or radiolabeled antibodies to detect the presence of drugs and other substances. False negative tests appeared to be common. Up until this time, the best known positive drug test from track and field involved U.S. discus thrower Ben Pluckett. His world record of 237 4", set July 1981 in Stockholm, was disallowed, and he was barred from international competition for life (a prohibition that has been commuted) because steroids showed up in one of his urine samples taken 5 1/2 months earlier at a meet in New Zealand.

In the 1983 PanAmerican Games held in Caracas, Venezuela, newly developed testing techniques were utilized and allowed for the testing of testosterone for the first time. These new methodologies employed the gas chromatography and mass spectrometry technology. Seventeen athletes from ten nations, including two from the United States, were disqualified from further competition (Almond 1984). Eleven athletes from the United States returned home rather than submit to testing.

The 1984 Olympic Games at Los Angeles, began the sophisticated methodologies currently utilized around the world. During the fifteen days of the Games, 1510 different urine specimens underwent 9400 screening analyses by a combination of gas chromatography, gas chromatography-mass spectrometry, and other procedures. These tests covered more than 200 different drugs and metabolites, including psychomotor stimulants, sympathomimetic amines, central nervous system stimulants, narcotic analgesics, and anabolic steroids (Catlin 1987). For the first time in the Olympic Games, Donike's testosterone/epitestosterone test for exogeneous steroids was employed.

After the conclusion of the Games, seven U.S. Olympic cyclists, including four medal winners, admitted that they had practiced *blood doping*. An eighth cyclist later stated that he also had a reinfusion of his own blood that had been drawn several weeks earlier. Verbal allegations claimed that these cyclists had participated in this doping under the direction of their coach because blood doping was not expressly defined on the prohibited drug list (Will 1985). Since that time, blood doping has been specifically added to the banned drug list.

In May 1987 a World Symposium of Doping in Sport was conducted in Florence, Italy, by the International Amateur Athletic Federation (IAAF), the world governing body for track and field, in conjunction with the International Athletic Foundation (IAF). Delegates were invited from all of the countries involved in international track and field competition. During this four-day meeting it became apparent that all countries in the world are experiencing problems with the misuse of substances perceived to enhance athletic performances (Official Proceedings).

In spite of all efforts of control and education, the 1988 Olympic Games in Seoul, Korea, presented more problems of drug abuse by athletes than at any previous competition, and the integrity of the Games is at an all time low.

A female swimmer from the United States was disqualified from the Olympics by testing positive for anabolic steroids in the pre-Olympic trials. However, nothing has shocked the international athletic movement as has the disqualification of Ben Johnson of Canada, after testing positive for anabolic steroids. His efforts and world record in the 100-meters had appeared to be almost superhuman, but ended in disqualification and removal of the record. His denial of drug use only sparked an investigation which has revealed a network of Canadian sprinter drug use. After the Canadian track team volunteered for squadwide testing in the wake of the Johnson scandal, two of its sprinters dropped off the roster. Questions as to how this could have happened will continue to be asked for a long time to come.

Two Bulgarian weight lifters tested positive for diuretics and the whole team withdrew and went home. The Hungarian weight lifting team also withdrew after two members of the team tested positive for anabolic steroids. This prompted a comment from an Olympic official that consideration should be given to removing weight lifting from the list of Olympic events.

In all, an unprecedented nine Olympians tested positive in Seoul, and were disqualified.

Other Problems and Action

It has become apparent that Olympic athletes are not the only ones involved in the abuse of performance enhancing drugs. On the afternoon of 19 October 1980 a world-class athlete, Augustinius (Stijn) Jaspers, was found dead in the upper bunk bed of his dormitory room at Clemson University. His death was baffling because he had been known to be in excellent condition. An autopsy revealed that Jaspers' heart was 31% larger than acceptable for a man of his size, and that a coronary artery on his left side was undersized. Although drugs were found in the apartment, they were not believed to be a factor in his death. However, further investigation revealed a sophisticated drug-traffic distribution system for dissemination of body enhancing substances to collegiate athletes (Brubaker 1980).

Jaspers' death was not the only one. Other deaths have included University of Maryland basketball star Len Bias, and Cleveland Browns safety Don Rogers. Both died from the toxic and adverse effects of cocaine, two years ago, within ten days of each other. Both were in the prime of their careers.

National attention was drawn to the medical problems caused by overuse of anabolic steroids in March 1984 when Daniel Baroudi, a twenty-six year-old body builder from Latrobe, Pennsylvania, died of liver cancer after having been on steroids for three years. He died three months after the initial diagnosis of the cancer, and lost almost eighty pounds prior to his death.

In April 1987 a West German heptathlete, Birgit Dressel, died of an immune system breakdown that reportedly was brought on by steroid abuse. This same year also brought the death of British cyclist Tommy Simpson (Goldman 1984). He was considered the best professional cyclist of his day. Toward the end of the thirteenth lap of the Tour de France, Simpson began to wander back and forth across the road. This lap involved a brutal 6,000 foot climb up a mountain in over 90-degree heat. He later collapsed in a coma and never recovered. A vial of methamphetamine was found in his pocket, and levels of the drug were found in his bloodstream on autopsy.

In October 1988 David Croudin, the special teams captain of the Atlanta Falcons Football Team, was pronounced dead after his wife called the paramedics because of his uncontrollable convulsions. Blood tests revealed extremely high levels of cocaine.

Consequently, amateur and professional athletic organizations have found it necessary to develop control measures like the international athletic governing federations have done. One such effort officially began at the 80th annual National Collegiate Athletic Association (NCAA) Convention held January 1986 in New Orleans. The NCAS established two policies concerning the use of drugs by student-athletes—Amendment 30 and Amendment 107. Amendment 30 spells out disciplinary actions and testing procedures. Amendment 107 provides for the financial costs of drug rehabilitation for athletes (Rovere 1986).

These positive actions have caught the attention of the athletes and the general public. It is now understood that an amateur student-athlete who chooses to use substances from the banned list will be tested and, if caught, disciplined, educated and rehabilitated. Testing is conducted at post-season events, national championships, and at bowl games.

The list of banned drugs falls into six categories: central nervous system stimulants, anabolic steroids, diuretics, substances prohibited for specific sports (e.g., beta-blockers), street drugs, and drugs having special consideration (e.g., blood doping, growth hormone, corticosteroids, local anesthetics, and drugs used for the treatment of asthma or exercise induced bronchospasm).

Professional Sports

Drug use is also rampant in professional sports. While many amateur sports have instituted mandatory drug testing, the professional player's unions have tried to forestall similar efforts with issues of privacy and civil liberties. However, increased efforts seem clearly warranted with the recent suspensions of NFL superstar players like Lawrence Taylor of the New York Giants and Dexter Manley of Washington, and NBA players such as Walter Davis of Phoenix and John Drew of Utah. In the last few years the major professional sports leagues have instituted drug policies that include testing for selected recreational or street drugs, but this drug testing should not be confused with the extensive prohibited drug listings of the amateur athletic federations.

The National Basketball Association has developed a drug policy that was supported by the player's union. The major premis of the program is to help people, rather than to drive them out of the league and into deeper desperation. The current policy states that any player convicted of, or pleading guilty to, a crime involving the use of heroin or cocaine, or who is found to have illegally used these drugs, is to be immediately dismissed from the league.

Such a player may apply for reinstatement after two years, but it requires the approval of both the Commissioner and the Player's Association. Any player who comes forward voluntarily to seek treatment for a drug problem is provided with the appropriate counseling and assistance under this program. The treatment is provided at the expense of the club, and the player continues to receive his salary without penalty. Any player who comes forward a second time for treatment is suspended without pay for the period of the treatment, but receives no further penalty. Any subsequent use of drugs, even if voluntarily disclosed, results in immediate and permanent dismissal from the NBA (Author's telephone conversation with NBA League Offices).

The National Football League utilizes an independent testing group which tests all players on each team during fall training camp. If any player tests positive for heroin or cocaine the first time, the results are not disclosed to the league. The results are disclosed to the club for which the athlete plays. A second positive test is disclosed to the league, and the player is suspended for a period of thirty days. A third positive test requires that the player be banned from the league for a period of one year, after which he may make application for reinstatement. Each application for reinstatement is handled on a case-by-case basis. It should be noted that the NFL began testing for anabolic steroids this year, but a positive test is not generally a punishable offense (Author's telephone conversation with NFL Offices).

Major League Baseball's policy leaves testing to the discretion of the Commissioner. If a player voluntarily comes forward concerning use of heroin or cocaine, he is not penalized and appropriate counseling and treatment is provided. Second offenses, or refusal to participate in testing, requires disciplinary action.

Types of Drugs

The factors involved in the athlete's selection of substances to obtain an advantage and those they choose to abuse are significantly varied. The only universal criterion is that a particular substance be purported to enhance his/her performance or relieve the post-competition stress. In general, there are three categories of drugs that appear to be specific to the athlete. These would include the *recreational or street drugs,* the *ergogenic drugs,* and the *performance continuance drugs.*

The recreational or street drugs include such drugs as alcohol, tobacco, marijuana, cocaine, and designer drugs (Zipes 1984). It appears there are various pharmacologic properties that may predispose a recreational drug for abuse. Although controversy exists as to these properties, some of them include: potential for fairly rapid development of tolerance, short duration of action, rapid onset of action, anticholinergic action, pleasurable euphoria, and a ritualistic administration (Woolley 1986).

The ergogenic drugs are those agents used by athletes for performance enhancement and body building. They generally fall into five divisions. These include: agents that make the person stronger, agents that make the body larger, agents that increase oxygen carrying capacity, agents that provide energy and/or stimulation, and agents that decrease recovery time after exertion. Most of these agents appear on banned drug lists and include: diuretics, antihypertensives, hormonal and steroidal compounds, growth hormone, glandulars, amphetamines and other stimulants (including caffeine), beta-blockers, designer substances, nutritional substances, and blood doping.

Performance continuance drugs include agents such as analgesics and anti-inflammatories. Nutritional supplements can also be included in this category. These supplements are as varied as the imagination. Some of these substances are bee pollen, amino acids, protein supplements, inosine, gammaoryzanol, octacosanol, herbal products, and complex carbohydrates.

Summary

Most experts are convinced the war on drugs in athletic competition will continue for a long time to come. As testing becomes more sophisticated so will the strategies to beat the tests. This can only lead to greater anxiety about the integrity of athletics. George Will, in a Newsweek editorial, stated:

> This anxiety is an institution in search of clarifying criteria. . . . Perhaps we are getting close to the key that unlocks the puzzle: techniques and technologies are unobjectionable when they improve performance without devaluing it. The use of certain exotic drugs or techniques alters the character of an activity and devalues it by making it exotic. . . . Sport is competition to demonstrate excellence in admired activities. The excellence is most praiseworthy when the activity demands virtues of the spirit—of character—as well as physical prowess. Admirable athletic attainments involve mental mastery of pain and exhaustion—the triumph of character, not chemistry, over adversity. We want sport to reward true grit, not sophisticated science. We do not want a child to ask an athlete, 'Can I get the autograph of your pharmacist?' (Wills 1985).

References

Almond, E.; Cart, J.; Harvey, R. (1984). Olympians finding the drug test a snap. *Los Angeles Times* Part III/Sunday, 29 January.

Beckett, A. H. and Cowan, D. A. (1979). Misuse of drugs in sport. *British Journal of Sports Medicine* 12:185–94.

Beckett, LA. H. (1981) Use and abuse of drugs in sport. *J. Biosoc Sci* Suppl. 7:163–170.

Brubaker, B. (1980) A pipeline full of drugs. *Sports Illustrated*.

Catlin, D. H.; Kammerer, R. C.; Hatton, F. K.; et al. (1987) Analytical chemistry at the Games of the XXIIIrd Olympiad in Los Angeles. *Clinical Chemistry* 33(2):319–.327.

Connolly, H. (1984) Fair play through drug tests? *Muscle and Fitness*. Feb. p. 90.

DiPasquale, M. G. (1984) *Drug use and detection in amateur sports.* pp. 16–18. Warkworth, Ontario: M.G.D. Press.

Donovan, J. E. and Jessor, R. (1983) Problem drinking and the dimension of involvement with drugs: A Guttman scalogram analysis. *Am J Public Health* 73:543–552.

Goldman, B. (1984) *Death in the locker room.* South Bend, Indiana: Icarus Press.

Hanley, D. F. (1979) *Sports medicine and physiology.* Philadelphia: W.B. Saunders Company.

Official Proceedings. (1987) *International Athletic Foundation World Symposium on Doping in Sport.* Florence, Italy. May.

Percy, E. C. (1978) Ergogenic aids in athletics. *Medicine and Science in Sports* 10(4):298–303.

Reedy, G. (1982) Drug abuse in sports: Denial fuels the problem. *Physician and Sportsmedicine* 10(4):114–123.

Rovere, G. D.; Haupt, H. A.; and Yates, C. S. (1986) Drug testing in a university athletic program: Protocol and implementation. *Physician and Sportsmedicine.* 14(4):69–76.

Schwartz, R. H. and Hawks, R. L. Laboratory detection of marijuana use. *JAMA* 254(6):788–792.

Strauss, R. H.; Liggett, M. T.; and Lanese, R. R. (1985) Anabolic steroid use and perceived effects in ten weight-trained women athletes. *JAMA* 253(19):2871–2973.

Taylor, W. N. (1984) The last word on steroids: Medicine can't ignore the issue. *Muscle and Fitness.* Feb. p. 88.

USOC Sportsmediscope (1988) 7(7):1.

Will, G. F. (1985) Editorial: Exploring the racer's edge. *Newsweek* 4 Feb. p. 88.

Woolley, B. H. (1983) Herbal pharmacology and toxicology. *J Collegium Aesculapium* 1(1):55–65.

Woolley, B. H. and Barnett, D.W. (1986) The use and misuse of drugs by athletes. *Houston Medical Journal* 2:29–35.

Zipes, J. S. (1984) Recreational mood altering chemicals. *Athletic Training.* Summer: p. 84–87.

CHAPTER 3

ETHICAL ISSUES OF DRUG USE IN SPORT

Ralph A. Vernacchia, Ph.D.

High-tech sport has redefined the concept of "fair play" as it relates to athletic training and performance. Traditional boundaries, once established and accepted by athletes and coaches, have been tested, stretched, and in some cases, violated in an effort to keep pace with the technological advances brought about by the increasing influence of science upon contemporary sport.

Traditional sport values which viewed success as a result of conscientious training, hard work, and sportsmanship predicated upon one's own best performance efforts, have been challenged and redefined by the arrival of the technosport concept. The world of sport has made tremendous use of technology, and much in sport is the product of technology (Eitzen and Sage 1986). Improvements in equipment, nutrition, and medical practices have certainly increased the training and performance capabilities of today's technologically influenced athlete. Along with these improvements have come the abuses, particularly the use of chemical substances to supplement the natural development of athletic talents. The use of drugs to enhance athletic training and performance, or in some cases to minimize the stress associated with athletic competition, are now a realistic choice for athletes who seek athletic excellence.

Fueled by the belief that competitive equality can only be achieved through the utilization of performance-enhancing substances, many elite athletes have adopted a variety of chemical and natural training procedures to ensure athletic success. Seduced by the lure of economic and political enticements, athletes have opted to override their values for the apparent promise of athletic success and fame. The advent of the *artificial athlete* has had a profound impact on the contemporary sporting world.

29

Faced with decisions testing their moral reasoning ability, athletes today are challenged to adhere to a high tech—high conscience ethic. It is the intent of this chapter to clarify the role of the athlete and coach in a technologically influenced athletic world which is in need of ethical reexamination. Sport and personal values, related to the outcomes of athletic training and performance, must be reevaluated by sport leaders and athletes if the integrity of the athletic experience is to be perpetuated and maintained. This chapter will explore the ethical considerations regarding drug use in sport from a philosophical, psycho-sociological, and leadership perspective.

This chapter is specifically directed towards bringing about a realization and understanding of the underlying social, economic, and political issues which are at the roots of the unethical and illegal drug related training and performance behaviors of athletes. Drug use in sport is thusly considered a symptomatic manifestation of a moral reluctance, upon the part of sport leaders and athletes, to comply and adhere to the traditional and contemporary athletic value orientations pertaining to fair and healthy athletic competition.

Psycho-Social and Philosophical Considerations

The following section addresses the influential psychological, sociological, and philosophical factors which effect the decisions and behaviors of administrators, coaches, and athletes as participants in the athletic environment. The understanding and realization of these existing factors upon one's moral decision-making abilities and the resulting behavioral choices are critical and may serve to illuminate the complexity of the problematic issue of drug use in sport. If we accept the fact an athlete's behavior is a product of his or her social environment, then we must make all efforts to understand and deal with this influential environment in a morally rational way.

Sport as a Microcosm of Society

Sport is a very powerful and visible social institution in many societies. Many of the social ills which plague society in general are magnified in the world of sport. Drug use and abuse in sport is a symptomatic manifestation of many underlying social and economic conditions which either positively or negatively affect the lives of every citizen.

In some ways, sport has served as a diversion from the problems society faces at large. Drug use in our society, whether utilized for medical, recreational, or coping purposes, is a reality. The United States is a drug nation. Besides being used for medical or therapeutic reasons, Americans utilize caffeine, nicotine, tranquilizers, alcohol, and illegal substances for a variety of personal reasons. Drug stores are found throughout our nation, and the pharmaceutical industry is a major economic institution. Powered by extensive advertising, the use of drugs is a major socially acceptable economic force in our society. Should we then be so appalled by the use of drugs in the sporting world?

In many cases athletes are unaware that their behavior is under the societal microscope and that their successes, as well as their failures, are evaluated according to godlike standards and expectations. The All-American image of the athlete is a traditional belief that still exists in our society, and sports are considered to be a socializing agent for the desired cultural values of our day. In many cases, the responsibility for modeling these values is a role which many athletes are either unaware of or unwilling to accept.

For these reasons we are shocked and appalled by the incidents of drug use and abuse among athletes. It is imperative that athletes at all levels understand their roles and responsibilities as they relate to their behavior on and off the field. This is where the coach's educational responsibilities reach far beyond the playing fields in order to develop, reinforce, and affirm a personal code of ethics for each athlete. In the long run, this educational charge is perhaps the coach's greatest responsibility when developing athletic talent. The coach must provide the ethical and moral leadership which is sorely needed to prevent drug abuse in sport.

Sport sociologist Harry Edwards described the existing relationship of sport and the American society as follows:

"Sports inevitably reflects the character of the larger society, particularly the ideological justifications people use to explain what happens in a society. American sports—the huge commercial enterprise Americans have made of both professional and amateur sports—tells us something important about our country: about what is happening to us as a nation and as a people. . . . The simple fact is that it is irrational for an athlete or a coach to behave ethically today. . . . That's true throughout our society: ends have utterly outstripped not only means but legitimate process itself. Sports is only the most visible manifestation of voracity that now characterizes all social relationships. . . . Athletes and sports institutions bear the brunt of people's general dissatisfaction with the ethical bankruptcy of their society." (Edwards et al. 1985, pp. 47, 48, 50)

In recent years the value orientation of sport has been closely scrutinized, evaluated, and challenged as a result of the ethically questionable behaviors displayed by athletes, coaches, administrators, and alumni. Evidence of morally misguided and unethical practices in the conduct of athletic programs abound in the media and, unfortunately, run the gamut from recruiting scandals to the sad reality of drug related deaths of athletes.

Such occurrences are certainly not commonplace in sport, but they do serve as symptomatic manifestations of serious underlying problems which can be best described as a *crisis of integrity* regarding the educational value of athletic programs.

Winning at All Costs

Given the relative importance societies place upon athletic excellence, it is important to examine the attitudes related to winning and success in sport. For many athletic participants and coaches, winning has become a passion in their lives. Unfortunately, this unchecked and intense passion can oftentimes lead to the development of obsessive attitudes and behaviors about the values and outcomes of athletic competition. In many cases, winning has become a counterproductive obsession in the lives of athletic administrators, coaches, and athletes.

Very few societal endeavors illustrate the achievement orientation of a nation than the collective sporting successes of their athletes. Former President Ford affirmed this concept in the following statement:

"Broadly speaking, outside of a national character and an educated society, there are few things more important to a country's growth and well-being than competitive athletics. . . . It has been said, too, that we are losing our competitive spirit in this country, the thing that made us great, the guts of the free-enterprise system. I don't agree with that; the competitive urge is deep rooted in the American character. . . . For one, do we realize how important it is to compete successfully with other nations? Not just the Russians, but many nations that are growing and challenging. Being a leader, the U.S. has an obligation to set high standards. I don't know of a better advertisement for a nation's good health than a healthy athletic representation. Athletics happens to be an extraordinary swift avenue of communication. The broader the achievement, the greater the impact.'' (Ford and Underwood 1974, p. 17)

As a microcosm of its societal values, the American sport model reflects the following orientation: success through competition; hard work; continual striving; deferred gratification; central values on societal progress; materialism; and external conformity (Eitzen and Sage 1986). Of all these values the concept of success through competition warrants closer examination in light of the present and future orientations and directions of sport.

Americans demand winners and heroes not only in sport but in many of our social institutions (e.g., politics, education, and religion). We honor winners and ignore the losers in sport. Young athletes soon learn that to the *victors belong the spoils,* including fame, social status, economic rewards, and other fringe benefits associated with athletic success. This product orientation soon outweighs the process by which these ends are achieved.

Sports have in many ways become a religion in American society. Athletes constantly seek perfection through their performances. They are asked to give a 110% effort in quest of superhuman performances, and may even be enshrined as legends in halls of fame if their efforts are deemed worthy. We are not very understanding or accepting of athletes whose performances reflect the human reality of their limited talents. We place a wide range of expectations and demands upon competing athletes in hopes of producing winners in whose glory and fame we can collectively and vicariously share.

It is apparent that the universal goal shared worldwide by athletes, governments, social agencies, and institutions—being number one— needs to be realistically and honestly re-evaluated. Physical educators, coaches, school administrators, and parents of athletes need to stress sports participation which encourages enjoyment, health, and personal self growth rather than ordaining winning as the prime objective of sport. This is not to rule out excellence in sport, but one should recognize that success is relevant to and dependent upon each person's capabilities, strengths, weaknesses, and limitations. If an athlete can be encouraged to give his or her best in athletic competition, then regardless of the outcome, that athlete can be considered a winner. The goal of athletics would then be to stress commitment to performance goals, development of skill through conscientious practice, and a determination to approach one's potential as an athlete through participation in sporting activities and athletic contests.

Fair Play and Cheating

The fair play concept of sport is the moral cornerstone upon which athletic training and competition is predicated. Sport participants engage in athletic contests with the belief that the rules which govern their training and performance efforts are equal for all competitors. Furthermore, sport participants subscribe to the belief their success or failure in the competitive setting is a direct result of the manner in which they skillfully and strategically employ their naturally developed athletic talents and abilities.

To intentionally violate this mutual trust among competitors is viewed as cheating. Training and competitive regulations are established and observed in order to ensure the performance integrity of each athlete, and considerable efforts are made to deal with rule violations in a just and expedient way. In some cases rules must be interpreted in light of the spirit of fairness by which they were formulated.

Each sport has an extensive set of absolute standards to govern and protect the fair play concept, but problems occur once these rules are applied to specific situations. It is the interpretation of rules and standards which tests the moral fiber and reasoning of administrators, coaches, and athletes. Sport participants are ethically challenged in many situations to acknowledge and adhere to the intent by which rules and standards of fair play have been formulated. The zeal and zest to excel and achieve winning performances oftentimes tempts the sport leader or participant to ignore or stretch the rules, leading to a *loophole* mentality which undermines the fair play orientation of sport. Such a mentality also encourages the use of unethical practices in sport by deeming them acceptable as long as they are not detected by officiating procedures or regulating sport agencies.

One of the most often misinterpreted concepts of sport is competition. We must recognize that competition in the athletic environment exists when an athlete or team is of equal ability with their opponent(s) or if the opponent possesses slightly greater or lesser ability than theirs. In many instances in sport this is not the case. For example, many coaches purposefully schedule weaker opponents to build the confidence of their teams as well as their won-loss record. Athletes are oftentimes placed in no-win or learning experience situations in which they are simply mismatched and/or overpowered by an opponent(s).

Once placed in such situations, coaches and athletes can soon become frustrated and seek a strategy or technique which can serve to make them competitive with their opponents. They no longer perceive their success as dependant upon their naturally developed skills and abilities, but upon strategies they can employ to defeat their opponent. It is at this point the coach and athlete are tempted to go beyond the rules to ensure success and turn to illegal training and performance enhancement measures to increase their competitive edge.

Even more disturbing is the fact that such learned competitive survival techniques may still be employed once the team or athlete has reached the top of their game. Athletes who follow this pattern tend to attribute their success to, and become dependant upon, the illegal techniques and substances which they utilized to achieve winning performances, rather than their naturally developed skill and abilities. If not regulated, participation and exposure to the competitive environment can spawn attitudes and behaviors which are certainly counterproductive to producing athletic excellence based upon the fair play sport ethic.

Power Orientation of Sport

It is an understatement to say today's athletes are bigger and stronger than their counterparts of even twenty years ago. Size and strength are prime prerequisites for athletic success, and all things being equal, the strongest and fastest performer will usually win out over the smaller, more skilled athlete. Athletes must possess a combination of power and skill to be effective in contemporary athletic arenas.

Athletes have either naturally or artificially attained a phenomenal degree of physical prowess which has gone far beyond the dimensions for which many sports were originally designed. As a result of this fact, the element of skill and strategy is being slowly eliminated from many sports. The rules for many sports were formulated during the mid to late nineteenth century and are now seemingly obsolete for the modern athlete.

Sports such as football, basketball, and baseball fall into this category. In all three of these sports, the athletes have far exceeded the original dimensions of the playing fields and the rules of the sport. Football is riddled by injuries created by powerful athletes who are restrained by the field's size and who are literally on a destructive collision course with each other. Add to this Astro Turf playing surfaces and equipment which gives the player a false sense of protection, and you have all the ingredients for a true battlefield environment.

Until recent rule changes in basketball (the three-point play and shot clock), the majority of play revolved around getting the ball to the big person for the high-percentage stuff shot. Action revolves around the power triangulation of the forwards and center, with occasional help from the penetrating guard. The 10-foot basket is seemingly becoming obsolete, especially for the collegiate and professional game. Many of the guards today are the same size as the centers of twenty years ago. There are very few highly skilled little men at the highest levels of competition.

Baseball pitchers are hurling the ball from a mound only sixty feet away. It is no wonder that the team that has the power pitchers usually has a distinct advantage. The batting averages of today's professional players can in no way justify their salaries nor match the averages of the great players of the past. Accusations of hopped-up baseballs and corked bats abound as players respond to performance pressures.

This scenario is true in many sports as athletes seek to keep pace with their opponents. The use of anabolic steroids is, of course, one of the main providers of increased size and strength which cannot be attained through training procedures alone. Power lifting has become an essential element for athletic success and in some cases—self-protection. Even though drug testing is utilized in performance situations, athletes are able to *chemically peak* themselves for athletic competitions. In some cases, athletic talent and prowess are no longer determined on the playing field or in the arena, but in a pharmaceutical laboratory.

Alienation Theory and Drug Use in Sport

Why do athletes take drugs to improve their performance in light of the long-term damage to their health? This is perhaps the most often posed question regarding drug abuse in sport.

The many financial and social rewards related to superior athletic performance, as well as social pressures and expectations, serve to create a value conflict in the athlete's mind. In an effort to settle this conflict, while at the same time remaining competitive with his or her peers, athletes have become alienated from their bodies.

Athletes soon learn to accept their bodies as a vehicle for athletic performance or success. In essence, the athlete uses his or her body as a means to obtain a desired outcome, thus detaching themselves from the ethical and health concerns which may impede their progress. The quest to gain the instrumental rewards of sport (money, fame, glory, records, championships, social status, scholarships, etc.) far outweighs the values associated with sport participation.

Athletes then hold the externalized perception they are forced to take drugs in order to remain competitive in their particular sport. Records and championships have become more important then their own health, and they relinquish the internal control of their bodies in light of these feelings. Their bodies become a tool to produce superior athletic performances. They think that they have but two choices: (1) take drugs to stay competitive, or (2) do not take the drugs and accept the fact that winning and records are no longer attainable goals (Coakley 1986).

In a recent article regarding drug use in sport, a United States shot-putter stated, "Drug taking is rampant. . . . Only the uninformed get caught. The pressure to take drugs is enormous. An athlete asks himself, 'Do I take drugs and win medals, or do I play fair and finish last?' " (Axtheim and Clifton 1988, p. 63).

Such feelings seem to offer support to the alienation theory of drug use in sport, as does the following statement by Al Oerter, a four-time Olympic champion in the discus throw:

> "When I returned to throwing from 1977 to '80 most everyone you talked to was using steroids or human growth hormone, and I even saw some guys getting a jolt of some dilute cocaine in a nasal spray before competition. I said, 'What happened to civility?' Here we have people changing personality a half hour before throwing. . . . You can't sit an athlete down and say, 'Work hard, and enjoy the improvement that *you* make. De-emphasize winning.' Even thoughtful people—though I don't understand it—find it necessary to win." (Moore 1988, p. 61)

Overtraining

Coaches and athletes alike have subscribed to the universal sport ethic of hard work as the main prerequisite for superior athletic performances. It is a widely accepted belief in the athletic world that the amount of an athlete's preparation and training is directly proportional to his or her performance outcomes. Although this belief may hold a general form of credibility, in sport it can oftentimes be overemphasized in the development of athletic talent. The general rule of thumb for the athlete is "the harder you work the better you'll be."

Such a concentrated approach to the development and performance of athletic skills can result in a very narrow view of the importance of athletics in one's life. The athlete may be encouraged to spend an inordinate amount of time in the training environment, to the point where they associate their identity solely with their training and performance outcomes. In many cases, athletes eventually come to realize that the athletic goals (realistic and unrealistic) to which they have totally devoted themselves are unattainable. This approach can be a disillusioning and embittering experience for athletes at all levels, especially if the educational, social, and economic aspects of their development have been neglected. There are an inordinate number of sport participants who sincerely believe they will become professional athletes, make an Olympic team, or be offered an athletic scholarship, etc. It is easy to understand how an athlete could turn to drugs to ease the pain associated with the disappointment of unrealized athletic dreams.

Several countries have selected to establish intensified and controlled training environments to ensure the performance effectiveness of athletes. These specialized environments are utilized to accelerate the training effect and ultimately result in superior athletic performances. Eastern European countries, namely Russia and East Germany, identify children who demonstrate a potential to perform athletically well at an early age. These children are then placed in state subsidized sports boarding schools specifically designed to develop their athletic abilities. The effectiveness of this procedure speaks for itself when one considers the athletic superiority these countries display in international athletic competitions such as the Olympic Games. Many Western countries are now following suit by the planned, systematic, and scientific development of athletic talent.

Such an approach for the development of athletic abilities is directly related to the economic ability of a nation to nurture the athletic talents of their athletes. Financial support for the development of athletic talent will usually result in better performances. To this end, the United States has relied on commercialization and the collegiate scholarship system to develop its talent pool for international competition. In essence, financially supported and specialized training procedures and environments are viewed as the determining factor in the cultivation of athletic talent.

This approach, in some ways, can be shortsighted in terms of the overall balanced social and educational development of the individual. It is this concentrated approach to athletic excellence which often leads to a distorted value orientation on the part of governments, sport leaders, and athletes. This practice can also be exclusionary, especially for those individuals and nations who wish to keep pace with training opportunities which may or may not be available as a result of their economic resources. For example, Third World countries can no longer participate effectively with the superpowers of international sport (Russia, East Germany, U.S., etc.). Is this practice fair to *all* competitors who participate in international sport? There appears to be a direct relationship between accessibility to the latest scientific and technological training methods and equipment and the economic vitality of individual athletes and/or their sponsoring agencies or governments.

Commercialism and Enjoyment of Sport

The 1980's has distinguished itself as the decade of the commercialized athletic performer. Prior to the 80's, athletes who received remuneration for their athletic performances were termed subsidized athletes. Commercialization has ended the era of the amateur athlete and ushered in the formal recognition of the professional athlete, especially in international athletics. Even the International Olympic Committee, the last bastion of amateur sport, has allowed professional athletes to participate in the Olympic Games. It is widely recognized that to participate successfully at the highest competitive levels of sport, athletes must seek external financial support to augment their training and travel.

Athletic prowess has become synonymous with economic success in the world of sport. Athletics are big business, and coaches, as well as athletes, seek considerable monetary remuneration for the promise of superior performance. Corporate and institutional sponsorship can aid athletes in their preparation for competition, but if not held in check it can strike at the foundations of sport participation for personal growth, the joy of competitive efforts, and the exhilaration of athletic success. Once the athlete becomes overly concerned or preoccupied with financial gain and security, his or her performance tends to be directed towards self-serving ends. Self-serving performances, initiated from the pocketbook rather than the heart, can lack humility and appear to dull the athlete's competitive and moral edge.

Performance and training enhancement drugs are attractive options for many athletes who elect to supplement their natural athletic talents, thus making them more financially marketable. The irony of this situation is that many athletes now demand appearance fees. They actually believe they should be paid for merely participating and showing up; their actual performances become secondary and are many times disappointing.

As stated previously, the health and legal risks associated with the use of these drugs are minimized in light of the promise and realization of financial gain and security. Soon sport takes on all the characteristics of work and loses its spontaneity, and athletes become driven to succeed for economic reasons rather than their love for the sport.

The cultivation of one's love for sport is perhaps the most enduring quality of sport involvement. Intrinsically generated sport performances, originating from the heart and reminiscent of a playful childhood, have always been the distinguishing characteristic of the most enjoyable and memorable athletic efforts for any individual.

This notion is best exemplified by the great Olympic champion Jesse Owens, who viewed running as a vehicle for physical freedom, individual expression, and as an activity from which he derived a sense of personal power. More importantly, he humbly described his love for running as follows:

> "I always loved running. . . . I wasn't very good at it, but I loved it because it was something you could do by yourself, and under your own power. You could go in any direction, fast or slow as you wanted, fighting the wind if you felt like it, seeking out new sights just on the strength of your feet and the courage of your lungs."
> (Baker 1986, p. 11)

Artificial and Natural Performance Enhancers

Until this point, the issue of drug use in sport has been directed towards the illegal or banned substances which athletes utilize to enhance their performance. There are several medical practices used by athletes to enhance their performance which cannot be detected or identified by testing procedures. Although many of these practices or training and performance aids may not be illegal, they may in fact give a distinct advantage to the athlete who utilizes them.

Artificial technological enhancement procedures employed by athletes include specialized athletic training programs, state-of-the art athletic equipment, and computerized training programs and skill analysis procedures. A variety of augmented training methods and procedures are now available to athletes which can facilitate the training effect.

The concept of artificial performance enhancement is not restricted to the athletic environment alone. For example, the concept of artificial intelligence is commonplace in many societies. The use of computers has been widely accepted and employed to help us keep pace with the demands of our technological world. Technologically sophisticated sport medicine practices have also been developed and employed to therapeutically treat athletic injuries. The sport sciences (e.g., exercise physiology, biomechanics, and sport psychology) have also successfully utilized technology to directly enhance the natural development of athletic talent and ability.

The point here is that the above-mentioned performance-enhancing methods are a by-product of acceptable evolutionary advances in the areas of sport technology and science. These practices are not considered illegal, but certainly give an advantage to the athlete who chooses to adopt such training and performance techniques. The question is, do they provide the user with an unfair natural advantage in athletic training and competition? The use of natural methods, such as altitude training, weight training, and plyometric training, are an acceptable by-product of research and experimentation in the sport sciences. Scientific advances have also led to the development of athletic equipment which has provided a distinct scientific edge in athletic competition. However, many athletes cannot financially afford to utilize such high-tech training procedures and equipment and thus may be economically excluded from this avenue for improving athletic performance.

There are several medical practices regarding performance enhancement which fall into the grey area of ethical appropriateness. These methods include blood doping, carbohydrate loading, growth hormone use, and electrical muscle stimulation, to name a few.

It can be argued these practices violate the spirit of fair play and the rules of competition because they can provide considerable performance advantages for the athlete. The use of these seemingly *natural* performance enhancers cannot be detected by testing procedures and are not considered illegal. The question is, are they morally and ethically illegal? This answer is relative to the individual interpretation of sport leaders and athletes and their respective value orientations toward sport.

The use of undetectable natural training and performance techniques may also be counterproductive to insuring the general health of the athlete. Such is the case of carbohydrate loading, which is a technique commonly employed by endurance athletes. Carbohydrate loading involves a practice by which an athlete completely depletes his or her

41

glycogen stores through an intense training session seven days prior to competition (Sherman 1983). During the next three days the athlete consumes only a protein-rich diet. For the remaining three days prior to competition, the athlete consumes a carbohydrate and sugar rich diet in an effort to maximize glycogen stores in the muscles. Since muscular contraction is ultimately glycogen dependent, the greater the availability of glycogen throughout an endurance event the more effective the athlete will be in prolonging and sustaining maximum athletic efforts.

This practice sounds both logical and harmless in theory, but what are the health-related implications of such a practice. First of all, the central nervous system needs carbohydrates to function properly, and for this reason, athletes who are in the carbohydrate denial phase tend to lack energy, muscular coordination, and can display listlessness, irritability, and depressed psychological orientations as well as mood swings. Three days of a low-carbohydrate diet can lead to hypoglycemia with associated nausea, fatigue, dizziness, and irritability (Sherman 1983). Injuries can also manifest themselves during this phase since muscular timing and coordination are minimally altered or affected. In the final stages of intense carbohydrate dietary infusion, the athlete's blood sugar levels rise dramatically and the athlete is energized and may display signs of hyperactivity, which can often prove to be counterproductive in the final resting stage prior to an intense endurance effort. The athlete tends to become anxious and can overtrain during this final stage in an effort to maintain self-confidence and to satiate the need for activity while in such an energized state. Are the physical and psychological states experienced by the athlete who employs such a natural training procedure, in fact, healthy? Do the training means justify the performance-enhanced effect of such a practice? Once again, these questions must be answered in light of the overall effect they will have upon the athlete's health. What are the short- and long-term effects of such training practices upon the athlete's health?

The rules of training and competition must be clearly specified in order to eliminate the confusion which now exists regarding the use of natural and other undetectable training practices. It is the responsibility of international and national sport federations to regulate and control the training and competitive environments in which their sports are conducted. These rules and regulations should be accompanied by a code of ethics for the coach and athlete. As it stands now, many of the unwritten rules' regarding sport are ambiguous and left to the individual interpretation of sport participants and officials.

Guidance is needed regarding the ethics of medical practices related to sport. A clear delineation needs to be made between the therapeutic use of drugs and the abuse of such methods when applied to healthy athletes who seek only to use such substances and practices solely to enhance their performance.

Recreational Drug Use

There are many substances classified as recreational drugs which do not directly enhance performance, but tend to be utilized by athletes as coping responses to the pressures of athletic training and competition. Winning and losing, as well as the role sport plays in the overall perspective of one's life, are very real concerns which add to the athletes susceptibility to the use of drugs. Without a balanced physical, intellectual, and moral orientation regarding the athletic experience, the athlete is surely on his or her road to disharmony regarding the role sport plays in their lives.

Athletes must learn to understand, recognize, and cope with the realities of the athletic world. It's not all fame and glory—the majority of athletic preparation includes sacrifice, personal setbacks, and struggle. Unless these realities are understood and kept in perspective by the athlete, he or she is certain to experience the disillusionment and embitterment which oftentimes leads to drug use. With guidance, athletes can learn to be in control of their behaviors. This can result from self-actualizing sport experiences generated and tempered by the reality of the athletic world and life in general.

Athletes who have lost control of their athletic and personal lives may lack the necessary foundational beliefs about the value orientation of their involvement in sport. In an effort to cope with the conflict which may arise from their athletic roles, they may tend to resort to the use of recreational drugs to ease the pressures of externally and internally induced goals and expectations. In many cases, athletes are not able to handle the diversions and rewards which accompany athletic fame and success.

The most abused and overlooked legal drug used by athletes today is alcohol. This is also the case for society at large. Athletes utilize alcohol for socialization purposes and to relieve the ritual and routine which accompanies the boredom of athletic training. Most often, however, athletes utilize alcohol to alleviate the uncomfortable pre- and post-competitive feelings of winning and losing. Other substances used to cope with these feelings and expectations are cocaine and marijuana. To even refer to these drugs as recreational implies a subtle acceptance of drug use as a coping response. We cannot, however, morally browbeat athletes into making appropriate decisions regarding their behaviors and responsibilities. We must appeal to their moral and ethical conscience, for the decision ultimately is theirs.

Drug Testing

Even though drug testing has been implemented to ensure fair competition, many coaches and athletes remain paranoid and skeptical regarding the ability of such measures to control the effects of drug use in the competitive setting. In order to alleviate these feelings, we need to institute controls for the training environment as well as for the competitive setting. Athletes have become extremely sophisticated in their ability to mask and regulate the use of performance-enhancing drugs.

Although athletes may test negative for drugs at the time of competition, they have learned to regulate their use during the training period so that their performance is undetectably enhanced. For this reason, if testing is to be used as a punitive deterrent to drug use, and is to be effective in protecting the fair play concept, then these tests must be implemented throughout the entire athletic training and performance cycle.

A lack of trust regarding the ability of athletes, coaches, and societies to self-regulate the drug problem now predominates the sporting scene as well as the public's perception. These feelings and perceptions are heightened when one considers the international sporting scene. The athletic Cold War between the Eastern European countries and many of the Western nations has certainly been escalated by the issue of drug use in sport. Perhaps an athletic summit between nations is in order to aid in the control of this problem, as well as to clarify the rules and roles sport should serve in contemporary societies throughout the world.

It is widely recognized that the problem of drug use in sport is beyond educational control, and that testing has become necessary to regulate and preserve the fair play concept in athletic training and competition. Drug testing is necessary because of the economic and political seductions in the athletic environment. In many cases, the perceived immediate gains of unethical medical practices in sport far outweigh the long-term moral and health consequences of such behaviors. One would prefer to combat the problem of drug abuse in sport solely with an educational approach affirming the appropriate value orientations of the athlete.

In reality, however, education and testing procedures must be employed—in concert—to bring about an effective change in the attitudes and behaviors of athletes and coaches.

Although many issues regarding the biological privacy of the athlete and the reliability of drug testing exists, drug testing can serve to eliminate the temptation to cheat or rationalize deviant behaviors on the part of the athlete and/or coach. Drug testing should be viewed as a necessary morality check on the ethical behaviors of athletes to protect and preserve the integrity of competitive athletics.

Traditional and Contemporary Values of Sport

The preceding section of this chapter dealt primarily with the social, economic, and political influences which tend to make athletes susceptible to drug use. This section will present a blend of traditional and contemporary values regarding sport in an effort to provide an ethical and moral decision-making framework for today's sport leaders and coaches.

The Classical View of Athletics and Olympism

Athletics played an integral part in the education of the Greek youth, who strove through sport to achieve a balanced personal harmony of the mind, body, and spirit. The Greeks exalted the good in man. Their pursuit of personal and athletic excellence reached its zenith during the Golden Age of Pericles, resulting in the establishment of a democratic society which was of the highest order.

This idealized educational philosophy was instrumental in the formulation of the Olympic games, which were initially conducted in 776 B.C. to honor the Greek god, Zeus. The ancient Greeks revered the athletes who, through athletic participation, sought to bring honor and glory not only to their nation and city-state, but most importantly, to themselves.

Greek athletes thoroughly enjoyed the challenge of the athletic contest. The effort put forth by the athlete to excel in athletic competition was the essence of the athletic experience. Material rewards were minimized since the athletes attempted to realize their physical and spiritual ideals through the discipline and sacrifice of training and the struggle of athletic competition. For the athlete the real prize was the honor of victory. The desire to excel and test his physical powers was the motive that turned the athlete's effort into joy (Gardiner 1978, p. 2).

The athletic ideals and values of the ancient Greeks were reviewed in 1896 by the French Baron Pierre de Coubertin, whose philosophy of *Olympism* forms the cornerstone of today's international Olympic Movement. In essence, the philosophy of Olympism is dedicated to the promotion of world peace through athletic activities (Douskov 1976).

Olympism is a philosophy which comprises the principles that contribute towards the perfection of man. It aims at a comprehensive upbringing of the individual leading to a harmonious development of the mental, physical, and moral faculties of the individual. The aims of the Olympic ideal are concerned with training and education, and the basic means of achieving these aims is systematic participation in exercise and sport.

The philosophical foundations of the Olympic Movement can serve as an inspirational guide for the examination, development, and establishment of sound values related to the objectives of athletic participation. Incorporation of Olympism-influenced objectives, pertaining to athletic participation, can provide guidance for contemporary athletic programs. These objectives include:

- Opportunities for broad-based participation in athletic programs and activities, or a sport-for-all orientation;
- An emphasis on altruism and humanism;
- Situational emphasis upon the development and testing of morals and ethics;
- A realization and understanding of the mind-body-spirit unity concept;
- The development of spirituality through the athletic experience;
- The clear establishment of the relationship between sport participation and educational enhancement;
- The promotion of personal, domestic, and world peace through athletic experiences;
- The development of an intrinsically oriented rationale for participation in sporting activities and contests based upon one's love of sport;
- An emphasis upon improvement through effort-conscious sport participation;
- The development and appreciation of one's expressive nature as a result of athletic participation;

- The development of self-discipline through training and performance related experiences;
- The honorable pursuit of athletic excellence.

It is the achievement orientation of athletics, the pursuit-of-excellence concept, which distinguishes it from sport and recreational endeavors. In its most classical form this orientation is best exemplified by the following phrase, which appears in the Homeric poem *The Iliad:* "... Always to be the best and excel over others." This was the exhortation of Peleus as he sent his son, Achilles, off to the Trojan wars in which Achilles ultimately won glory and lost his life (Douskov 1976).

The Olympic Ideal

According to the Olympic ideal, the pursuit of athletic excellence is to be balanced, complemented, and realized by placing equal emphasis upon the intellectual, spiritual, social, and ethical growth and development of the aspiring athlete.

Ultimately, the athlete must evaluate how he or she achieved success and recognition, for there is a distinct difference between a winner and a champion. Champions are remembered and valued not solely for what they achieved but how they earned their recognition, and in some cases, how they responded in defeat. Although there are many winners in athletics, there are truly only a few champions. The champion is humble and compassionate in victory, dignified in defeat, and resolved to be the best in future competitive situations.

The achievement orientation of sport administrators, coaches, and athletes should reflect their desire to be winners and champions, while at the same time realizing that although one cannot always win, they can always attain the satisfying self-actualizing benefits of a championship effort. It is, therefore, the educational charge and challenge of both coaches and athletes to achieve *victory with honor.*

It is also important to note that the very elements of overcompetition, specialization, and professionalism which caused the downfall of the ancient Olympic Games have manifested themselves once again in the modern Games. As the Olympic Movement, and athletics in general, progress into the twenty-first century, their greatest challenge would seem to be the application of traditional values, formulated during an industrial age, to sport as it now exists in the highly technological world.

Drug usage and unethical medical practices are rampant in international and professional sport and must be policed and abolished. Athletes

and coaches must speak out against such practices, create a global awareness of this problem, and condemn such practices as unethical and im-
moral. We are slowly extracting the natural element from athletics at its
highest levels, and soon we will be left with technologically developed
and medically primed athletes who have been politically and economically socialized to sacrifice their long-term health for the short-term
gratification of athletic success. Today's athletes are often challenged to
override their social, moral, and ethical consciences in favor of the personal gain resulting from athletic success and fame.

A reexamination of the role ethics plays in the medical aspects of
national and international sport is sorely needed. Sports medicine
authorities must establish and implement sound guidelines aimed at
protecting the athlete's long-term health while denouncing the unethical
medical practices now becoming commonplace in sport.

The modern athletic world could be well served if it would reflect
upon the traditional values of sport related to the formulation of contemporary athletic training and performance techniques and strategies. It is
true that the technological advances of our day have brought about significant societal progress, but we must keep in mind, however, that
change for the sake of change does not necessarily result in improvement
or progress in a society. The same is true of the athletic world.

It is attractive to be myopic about the immediate performance gains
which can be realized in performance as a result of technological and
chemical innovations, but our challenge will be to create an awareness of
the long-term ramifications of our decisions as they relate to the health
and well being of the athletic participant, as well as to the future of competitive athletics.

Leadership

Leadership is at the hub of the athletic experience and is the most
important component of any athletic program if ethically and morally
sound goals and behaviors are to be realized. For this reason, administrators and coaches must possess and demonstrate a commitment to
the foundational beliefs which govern the conduct of their programs.
More importantly, it is the responsibility of sport leaders to openly trans-
mit these beliefs to the participants who strive for athletic excellence
under their guidance.

Before athletes are required to comply with the rules and regulations of their sport, sport leaders and parents must have their moral houses in order. This is particularly true of administrators and coaches since they have a profound influence upon the attitudes and behaviors of their charges. They should have a clearly defined philosophy which emphasizes the moral and ethical environment in which athletic training and competition are conducted.

The challenge for the sport leader is not only to provide the rhetoric of sound foundational beliefs regarding the value and ethics of athletic participation, but to demonstrate these beliefs at the appropriate time in order to give an educated and experiential perspective to the world of athletics. Sport leaders must clearly understand the influence and responsibilities of their positions and act accordingly, for as the adage states, "The apple does not fall far from the tree." We must seek stability in sport through foundational beliefs and behaviors which serve as a guiding influence for the athlete, whose successes and failures require cultivation to reach fruition.

In many cases the term "athletic excellence" has been synonymous with winning. Although the final outcome of athletic competition can be easily and objectively measured by performance outcomes, we must also balance this orientation with the subjective measures by which these outcomes are attained. As stated previously, how athletic excellence is achieved is as important as what is achieved. A process orientation to sport participation must also be identified to add substance, integrity, and validity to the quest for athletic excellence.

Programmatic Goals and Values

Concerns of athletic programs should center about the creation of community and the primary relationships among participants as a result of participation in *active sport* experiences. Such experiences are directed towards rejecting the notions of passive recreation, consumption, and spectatorship in favor of active sport for fitness and recreation. Programmatic emphasis would also be placed upon: individual expressions above group conformity; self-discipline above authority; independence above dependence; and the moral reasoning and decision-making ability of the athlete regarding the integrity of their behaviors as they relate to the performance outcomes they seek.

The *process* approach to athletic participation recognizes competition for its own pleasure, not to generate conditional self-worth or role specific relationships, and is resistant to the development of a self-perception which is solely dependent upon excellence derived and related to competitive merit. A process orientation to sport also gives preference to cooperation over competition and emphasizes skill development in lifetime activities for preventative health. In such an orientation, extrinsic and comparative forms of reward are replaced with intrinsic forms of reward, which are personally satisfying and primarily self-actualizing. Thus, the utilitarian and competitive nature of sport can be kept in perspective by sport participants and leaders alike.

School-centered programs are encouraged for the implementation and realization of an educationally based athletic program, primarily to control and regulate the quality of the sporting experience. However, this concept is undergoing serious reevaluation because of the financial strain athletic programs face in light of budgetary concerns related to the funding of athletics at all levels. For this reason, many contemporary athletic programs have been overly concerned about the revenue-producing capabilities of sport, while at the same time ignoring the ethical and moral implications of such an approach. At the higher levels of athletics (university and international levels), the professional or corporate sport model has been adopted in an effort to economically survive the funding pressures and, in some cases, has replaced the educational model upon which many athletic programs were established.

In an educational athletic model, the leader's primary function is to assist his or her followers in attaining predetermined goals which are mutually agreed upon. These goals are athlete oriented, and the leader serves to facilitate their realization and attainment, as opposed to utilizing methods which are manipulating, coercive, and appeasing for the purpose of shaping appropriate behavior.

Coaches should be viewed as resource persons and advisors rather than authority figures. Humanistically oriented coaches establish an empathic identification with their athletes, an openness to the athletic experience, and a commitment to develop a positive self-concept in others via sporting activities. The ultimate leadership challenge for coaches is to develop athletes who make their own decisions, are self-reliant, and are responsible and accountable for their own behavior.

The Coach's Role and Responsibilities

Of all the sport leaders, the coach is the most influential in determining and influencing the athlete's values, attitudes, and behaviors. The coach must wear many hats and serve many roles in the development of an athlete's moral, physical, spiritual, and emotional development. For the athlete, the coach is a leader, role model, disciplinarian, friend, counselor, parent substitute, and family member. For the parent, the coach is a provider of fair and equal opportunity to their child. The coach can make or break the sporting experience because "the athlete and athletics meet at the coach" (McGuire 1986).

The coach has a specific responsibility to contribute to the physical, moral, spiritual, and emotional development of the athlete through his or her interactions with young persons via athletic participation. The developmental charge of the coach revolves around the recognition and employment of clearly defined foundational beliefs in the dynamic educational environment of athletics.

The coach is charged with tempering the athlete's passions and zeal for achieving athletic excellence. It is the coach who has the privilege of establishing an impressionable educational bond with the athlete. Over time and through considerable sacrifice and dedication to a common goal, the athlete learns to trust and respect the coach. The coach serves to guide and protect the athlete throughout his or her athletic experience. The quality of this experience has strong implications in terms of the future attitudes and behaviors of young people, both on and off the athletic field.

Athletics can be a very influential training ground for the moral reasoning and subsequent personal decision-making capabilities of the coach and athlete alike. Absolute values, which all sport leaders and participants recognize and verbally agree to uphold, are tested as a result of actual athletic training and competitive experiences. It is within these situational experiences that the moral and ethical maturity of the coach must be activated to ensure the athlete's compliance with previously and mutually agreed upon foundational beliefs regarding athletic and personal behavior.

Summary

In the final analysis, the ethical issues regarding drug use in sport revolve around the athlete's moral reasoning ability. This ability is derived from a clear awareness and understanding of the true meaning and value of sport involvement. Athletic ideals are transmitted by words, actions, and deeds of sport leaders, whose responsibility it is to establish an ethically sound athletic environment.

In the purest sense, drug use to enhance performance or to deal with the pressures of athletic competition has no place in sport. Administrators, coaches, parents, and athletes must work in concert to raise and constantly reinforce the athletic conscience and ideals of sport participants, who may be challenged to ignore, minimize, or override their personal values. We must encourage all persons involved in sport to demonstratively accept the challenge of pursuing athletic excellence in an honorable fashion.

References

Axtheim, P. and Clifton, T. (1988) Using chemistry to get the gold. *Newsweek.* 25 July.

Baker, W. (1986) *Jesse Owens, An American life.* New York: The Free Press.

Coakley, J. J. (1986) *Sport in society: Issues and controversies.* 3rd ed. St. Louis: C. V. Mosby Co.

Douskov, I. ed. (1976) *The olympic games.* Athens, Greece: Ekdotike Athenon S. A.

Edwards, H. et. al (1985) Sports: How dirty a game. *Harper's Magazine.* 271(1624) Sept.

Eitzen, S. and Sage, G. (1986) *Sociology of North American Sport.* 3rd ed. Dubuque, Iowa: Wm. C. Brown.

Ford, G. and Underwood, J. (1974) In defense of the competitive urge. *Sports Illustrated.* 41(2) July.

Gardiner, E. N. (1978) *Athletics of the ancient world.* Chicago: Ares Publishers, Inc.

McGuire, R. (1986) The coach—someone special. In *Coaching mental excellence: It does matter whether you win or lose.* R. McGuire, D. Cook, and R. Vernacchia. The Athletics Congress Coaching Certification Manual, Level II.

Moore, K. (1988) Old men and the discus. *Sports Illustrated.* 69(4) July.

Sherman, W. M. (1983) Carbohydrates, muscle glycogen, and muscle glycogen supercompensation. In *Ergogenic aids in sport* ed. M. Williams, Champaign IL: Human Kinetics Publishers.

Suggested Readings

Morgan, W. J. and Meier, K. V. eds. (1988) *Philosophic inquiry in sport,* Champaign IL: Human Kinetics Publishers. (See Part IV *Sport and ethics,* which presents essays on competition, sportsmanship, cheating, and failure—as well as drugs and sports.)

Chapter 4

ANABOLIC-ANDROGENIC STEROIDS

James E. Wright, Ph.D.

Interest and participation in physical activities and sports have in-creased tremendously over the past several decades. Among the many reasons for this are the increased availability of leisure time, facilities, equipment, and information on how to exercise and on the mental and physical benefits of physical training. Developments in electronics and communications technology have helped bring sports into everyone's living room. These and other factors have altered the traditional role of sports in society. From a pleasant past time, athletics as never before has the potential to become a profession, a business, and a part of life which can dramatically change one's social, as well as financial, status. These factors are central among the many which are inspiring countless in-dividuals of all ages to "go for the gold."

Unfortunately, the winner-take-all pattern of compensation and notoriety has in turn prompted a win-at-all-costs philosophy among many athletes and coaches. A number of top athletes have even publicly stated that they would use any means at their disposal, even if it meant risking serious illness or death, to win. The decision, "at what price, victory?" places the athlete, coach, trainer, medical personnel, administrators, and even parents in precarious positions, particularly with respect to the use of drugs to alter mental or physical states, or performance.

The use of drugs is not new. They have been a feature of human life in all places on the earth and in all ages of recorded history. The use of substances thought to enhance physical work capacities, known as er-gogenic aids, dates back thousands of years. The use of drugs in athletics, however, has more recently been scrutinized from the idealistic philosophical perspective on which the modern Olympic Games was

53

founded in 1896—that the overriding objective is not to win but to take part.

It is well accepted that ergogenic drugs are extensively used at virtually all levels of competition in a wide variety of athletic activities. Many factors have contributed to this drug use (Figure 1). One major reason for an increase in the use of drugs, such as the anabolic-androgenic steroids (AS), has been the controversy over the interpretation and applicability of medical and scientific studies of their effects. One of the principal physiological actions of AS is their stimulation of a *constructive* phase of metabolism, a build up of protein in the body. Much of the theoretical basis for their application in both clinical medicine and sports is derived from this attribute, particularly because proteins make up the basic structural, contractile, and enzymatic components of muscle tissue, as well as serving as precursors of various hormones and energy conveyors (adenosine triphosphate, and creatine phosphate). Despite the several thousand research studies, problems and disagreements arise with regard to the organs, tissues, and extent to which this anabolism (protein buildup) is manifested under various conditions particularly in athletics, and in any resulting long- or short-term physical, physiological, or psychological effects. This review is intended to provide an overview of primarily the short-term effects of AS on physique, physiological and performance functions, and health risks; and to raise questions that must be answered if society is to come to grips with the growing use of AS in athletics.

By definition, AS are a class of synthetic compounds which closely resemble testosterone, the male sex hormone. Testosterone, which begins to be secreted in quantity by the testes at puberty (a 20 to 40-fold increase over early childhood levels), is largely responsible for the differences in muscle, bone structure and density, fat mass and distribution, in the organs, systems and physical (skin, hair, voice, etc.) and behavioral characteristics that distinguish males from females. Testosterone is called an androgen, a term derived from the Greek word meaning *male producing*. However, it is also very anabolic in that it strongly stimulates the retention of nitrogen and the buildup of body protein.

As the fields of steroid biochemistry and pharmacology developed from the 1930s through the 1960s, scientists met with some success in chemically modifying the structure of the testosterone molecule to produce anabolic steroids that elicit positive effects on muscle and body protein metabolism at dose levels which *tend* not to increase other virilizing characteristics. However, no *purely anabolic* steroid has yet been

54

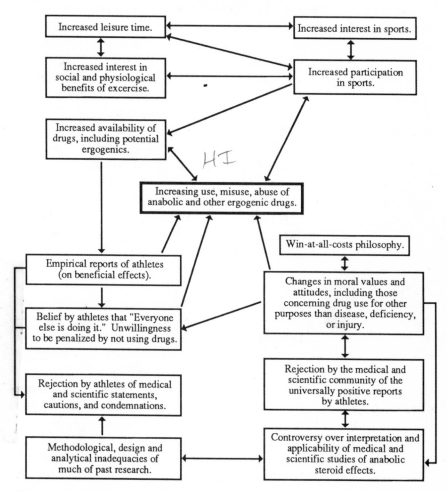

Figure 1. Influences on AS use in athletics.

developed. All available drugs exhibit both types of activities, but to varying degrees in different conditions and individuals. As Kruskemper (1968) has stated, the anabolic effects differ from the androgenic only in location and not in essence. There are a couple of dozen different AS currently available for administration in pill form or by injection, some examples of which appear in Figure 2.

Soon after their introduction, AS began to be used in a wide variety of medical conditions, perhaps to the extent that the rationale for their therapeutic use occasionally became questionable. This impression was supported by the fact that much of the data on the actions of these drugs were obtained from uncontrolled clinical trials. However, the amount of data from controlled investigations is considerable, and that of positive observations collected in poorly or uncontrolled studies is too voluminous to be ignored. Most comprehensive clinical and biochemical reviews conclude that there is convincing evidence on the usefulness and effectiveness of AS in the treatment of a variety of disorders (Kochakian 1976; Kopera 1985; Kruskemper 1968).

The most obvious clinical use is as replacement therapy for hypogonadal men. AS are the best nonspecific stimulants of erythropoiesis and thus are widely used in the treatment of anemias, including hypo- and aplastic, hemolytic anemia, anemias due to renal failure and to irradiation and the use of cytotoxic drugs, and in myeloid metaplasia, lymphoma and leukemia (Kopera 1985). AS are effective in the management of autosomally dominant hereditary angioneurotic edema. AS have also been used for palliative therapy in breast carcinoma (Turner 1981) and advanced osteoporosis (Dequeker and Geusens 1985). Growth hormone is also the treatment of choice for the various forms of stunted growth. Such therapy is very expensive and effective, although careful dosing and observation of patients are required to reduce the risk of too rapid acceleration of bone maturation with adverse effects on ultimate height. AS have also been used therapeutically in cases of malnutrition, certain soft tissue injuries, and wasting diseases (Kruskemper 1968).

AS are only one group of compounds which share the characteristic four-ring steroid skeleton. They should not be confused with other types of steroids, such as the glucocorticoids, an example of which is cortisol, which is produced by the adrenal gland and which affects metabolism in a negative (catabolic) manner but which also acts to reduce inflammation. Both oral and injectable preparations of anti-inflammatory steroids have many effects on body and protein metabolism opposite to those of the

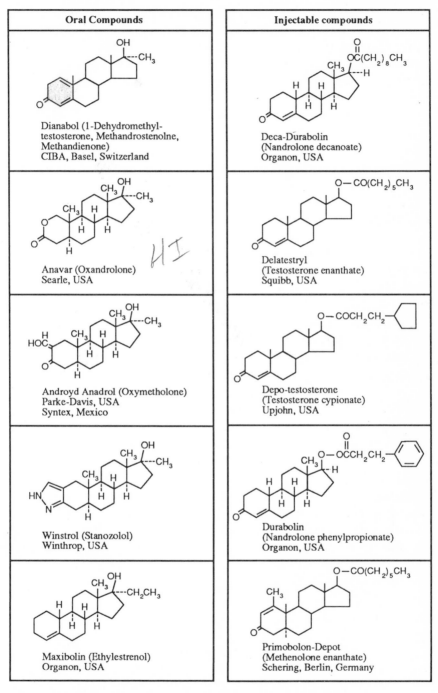

Figure 2. Examples of some anabolic-androgenic steroids.

AS. The structural similarities between the two groups, however, lead to some similar adverse effects, most notably on the liver (Orlandi and Jezequel 1972) and psyche (Alcena and Alexopoulos 1985; Byyny 1976; Lewis and Smith 1983; Pope and Katz 1988; Tennant, Black, and Voy 1988).

Many experiments have been carried out to assess the actions and health and performance effects of AS. Because of their general physiological and biochemical similarities to humans, and because the results of many well-designed and conducted animal studies are relatively conclusive on the specific issues and questions they have addressed, much can be gleaned from the animal research. Perhaps most valuable in this regard have been the initial and/or confirmatory findings of the various adverse effects. The majority of studies using animals, including a variety of rodents, dogs, cats, monkeys, and domestic farm animals, have been unable to demonstrate in normal healthy males consistent positive effects on lean body mass or performance variables exceeding those which would result from exercise alone. However, animals deficient in natural anabolic hormone levels (relative to young males), such as castrated males, females, and old animals, often do show substantial increases in muscle mass with AS administration.

The question of whether AS actually do affect muscle size and performance capacities, and to what extent, cannot be answered conclusively at this time based on the 40-or-so studies which have been published in scientific journals in the last quarter century. The reasons for this lack of consensus are numerous and complex (Table 1). Despite the inconsistencies that have been pointed out (Ryan 1976; O'Shea 1978; Wright 1978 and 1980; Wilson and Griffin, 1980; Haupt and Rovere 1984; Lamb 1984; Wilson 1988), it would appear that the more anabolic forms of exercise, such as conventional strength training and bodybuilding, does facilitate increases in body mass.

Table 1. Reasons for Lack of Consensus on AS Effects on Health and Performance Variables.

Subjects	The number of subjects, their experience in weight used training, and physical condition at the start of the study varied.
Diet	Most not controlled or recorded.
Training programs	Volumes and intensities varied.
Testing programs	Strength often not measured in the training mode. Body composition often assessed from skinfold estimates. Health effects often mismeasured (not organ specific) or not measured.
Drugs	Variable, and few have reported on athletes self-administering multiple drugs.
Study	Some crossover, some single blind, some double blind, some not blind, some no controls.
Drug mechanisms of action	Unknown and varying degrees of anabolic, anticatabolic, and motivational effects depending upon the circumstances.
Dosages	Variable, only two studies administered dosages approximating those currently used by competing athletes.
Length of study	Variable and generally short; very few have reported on prolonged training and AS self-administration.
Placebo effect	Well documented for most drugs; yet most data suggest that athletes can readily defeat. As administration making it virtually impossible to conduct blind studies.
Data interpretation	Variable, dependent upon the background and experience (scientific, clinical, athletic, administrative), general perspective, and goals of interpreters.
Legal and ethical issues	Preclude design and execution of a well-controlled study, using doses and patterns of administration of drugs with potentially fatal effects in healthy volunteers and in a manner comparable to that currently used by competitors.

An adequate diet also seems to be a critical ingredient in producing this effect, although *adequate,* much the same as with training volume and intensity, has yet to be defined with regard to the intake of any specific dietary component (protein, carbohydrate, vitamin, mineral or other nutrient, or overall caloric intake). In no study were fat and caloric intake controlled, and little mention was made of vitamin-mineral supplementation and protein intakes, which were probably lower than those of most serious bodybuilders.

The effects of AS on body composition are less clear, although there appears to be a reduction in the percentage, if not the absolute quantity, of body fat. These changes resulted primarily from the increase in body weight as there were not consistent reductions in skinfolds. Studies designed to determine how diet interacts with AS and training to effect body composition have not been conducted.

Individuals experienced in weight training, and who continue training during AS administration, seem to consistently increase their strength over what would have been expected (i.e., as observed in controls) from training alone. In the vast majority of studies reported, subjects given AS, but not pre-trained with weights, did not tend to gain more strength than did the controls.

The reasons for this difference between experienced and inexperienced subjects remains speculative, much as do the differences between the empirical observations and self-reports of many athletes and coaches, and what has been reported in the scientific literature. AS are known to have both anabolic and anticatabolic, as well as placebo, effects and they probably also influence motivation. The anticatabolic effects are probably the more important in explaining the differences noted above. In this respect, AS can convert a negative nitrogen balance to a positive one by improving the utilization and retention of injected protein (Goodman and Gilman 1975; Kruskemper 1968; Kochakian 1976), and they can reverse the catabolic effects of administered synthetic, as well as natural, corticosteroids that are released in times of physical or emotional stress (Dahlman, Widjaja, and Reinauer 1981; Kruskemper 1968; Morano 1984), this latter effect being dependent upon intake of an adequate quality and quantity of protein (Kruskemper 1968; Kochakian 1976). This reversal of protein catabolism has been shown to last for the duration of AS treatment, but the induced positive nitrogen balance eventually returns to an equilibrium as a result of homeostatic mechanisms which work to maintain nitrogen balance in the normal state. In normal healthy humans and animals, i.e., those who are *unstressed* and have normal levels of testosterone, the anticatabolic effects do not come into play, and the anabolic effects are generally small and short-lived.

The reason AS are called anabolic is that they cause an increase in protein synthesis in target tissues. AS increase protein synthesis through their interactions with specific receptor proteins within their target tissues, which include skeletal and heart muscle, skin, testes, prostate, and brain. These hormone-receptor complexes interact in turn with receptor sites on the chromosomes which elicit gene transcription and the subsequent synthesis of messenger RNA, and ultimately various proteins (Figure 3).

Although all skeletal muscles respond to androgens, there is a considerable inter-species variation in the sensitivity of individual muscles and muscle groups to anabolic steroids. In man, the muscles of the pectoral and shoulder girdle appear to be most sensitive (Wilson and Gloyna 1970). The limiting factor, with respect to AS effects, appears to be the number of existing AS-receptor complexes. Although muscle hypertrophy results in an increased number of unsaturated receptors (Hickson et al. 1983), as does an increase in estrogen levels (Rance and Max 1984), exorbitant doses of AS have no further effect on muscle once receptor saturation is achieved. This is thought to occur at close to normal androgen levels in healthy adult males (Wilson 1988). Even though the mechanism by which growth is promoted is not understood, the effect of the anabolic process in skeletal muscle is to induce the formation of new myofilaments and the division of enlarging myofibrils (Venable 1966).

The AS associated body weight increases could be due to still other mechanisms. In addition to nitrogen, AS reduce the amounts of potassium, phosphorus and calcium, and to some extent sodium and chloride, lost in the urine. In two studies, the amount of potassium and nitrogen retained after six weeks of 100 mg per day of methandrostenolone as disproportionately large for the increase to have been *normal* muscle (Hervey et al. 1976; Hervey et al. 1981). Some weight gain is probably due to increased sodium retention which can occasionally be substantial (Kochakian 1976; Kruskemper 1968). AS given in pharmacological doses increase hemoglobin and hematocrit substantially (Alen 1985), and may increase total blood volume by 15 percent or more (Holma 1977). Weight changes correlated well with blood volume changes in one study (Holma 1977), and it has been suggested that in those who do experience increased blood volumes, the effect on athletic performance might be similar to that achieved by the practice of blood doping in some sports (Puffer 1986). Despite these changes and those anti-catabolic effects pre-

61

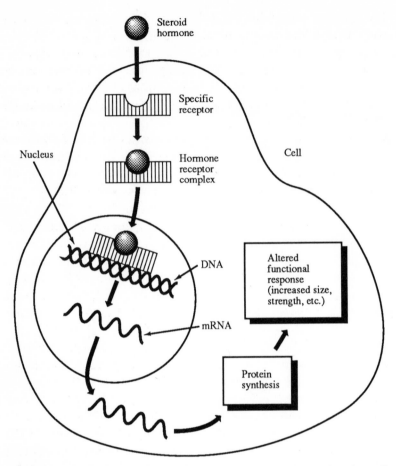

Figure 3. Schematic representation of the mechanism of action of steroid hormones.

viously discussed that would theoretically be expected to facilitate increases in training volume and/or intensity and to improve cardiorespiratory capacities, the studies reported to date have been unable to document consistent significant improvements in aerobic power (predicted or measured maximal oxygen uptake) or performance (Haupt and Rovere 1984; Lamb 1984; Wright 1980). However, as in the case of the weight training studies, the research published to date is not conclusive. A study of appropriate length and design has yet to be conducted.

The third mechanism by which AS might affect lean mass, exercise capacities, and performance is through the nervous system. Androgen receptors occur in both the brain and in alpha motor neurons (Sar and Stumpf 1977; Stumpf and Sar 1976) whose size and number can be strongly influenced by AS (Arnold 1984; Kurz et al. 1986). Androgens have been implicated in facilitating the release of acetylcholine at the neuromuscular junction (Vyskocil and Gutmann 1977) and in elevating monoamine levels in the central nervous system. Electroencephalographic recordings of subjects given a wide range of doses of AS mimicked those seen when amphetamines and tricyclic antidepressants were given (Itil 1976; Itil et al. 1974). It is commonly believed and reported by athletes that they *feel* more energetic and aggressive, and that they can train longer and harder when using AS (Strauss et al. 1983), and, in fact, these and other effects are sufficient to make it difficult to conduct a truly blind study (Freed et al. 1975; Wilson 1988). Although both the relative contribution and the specific mechanism are not known, it seems reasonable to assume that AS effects on the nervous system could contribute significantly to any changes in exercise capacities or performance.

The role of AS in the etiology of various diseases is unclear at present. However, in both animals and humans, in therapeutic trials and in laboratory studies, AS use has been associated with numerous deleterious changes in risk factors and in the physiology of sundry organs and body systems which suggest the potential for subsequent health problems (ACSM 1984; Kruskemper 1968; NSCA 1985; Wright 1980). The best documented effects include those on the liver, cardiovascular, and reproductive systems; although effects on the nervous system, psyche, and behavior (Annitto and Layman 1980; Feinhar and Alvarez 1985; Itil 1976; Itil et al. 1974, Pope and Katz 1988) and other miscellaneous changes (ACSM 1984; Kochakian 1976; Kruskemper 1968) may also have a significant impact on health.

Some demonstrated effects of exogenous male homrones that may affect the development of cardiovascular disease include: hyperinsulinism and altered glucose tolerance (Cohen and Hickman 1987) changes in lipoproteins fractions (Hurley et al. 1984; Webb et al. 1984), triglyceride levels (Olsson et al. 1974) concentration of several clotting factors; elevations of blood pressure (Freed et al. 1975; Salgado and Selye 1954) and in animals, changes in the myocardium itself (Appell et al. 1983; Behrendt 1977; Behendt and Boffin 1977). Cerebrovascular accidents have been reported in several patients using AS (Nagleberg et al.

1986; Schiozawa et al. 1982). It should be noted, however, that although these effects may vary for different individuals and situations, all of the above effects, except changes in the myocardium (which have not been followed), have been demonstrated to be fully reversible within a period of several months following cessation of use.

Liver structure and function have likewise been altered by administration of AS. Structural changes have been observed in both humans (Orlandi and Jezequel 1972; Schaffner et al. 1960) and animals (Stang-Voss and Appell 1981; Taylor et al. 1982). Changes in transminase levels, alkaline phosphatase, bilirubin, and increased sodium bromosulphophthalein (BSP) retention have all been reported on numerous occasions (Sherlock 1979) reflecting an impaired excretory function. The cholestasis has progressed to jaundice (Peters et al. 1958; Schaffner et al. 1959) and been fatal in some cases (Kruskemper 1968). Peliosis hepatis has been observed in a variety of clinical circumstances in which AS were utilized (Asano et al. 1982; Bagheri and Boyer 1974), as have liver tumors (Ishak 1981; Paradineas et al. 1977), with one fatal case in a bodybuilder (Overly et al. 1984). The cause-effect relationships between AS and the above occurrences is strengthened by the return of normal blood values and excretory function, the regression of tumors, a general recovery, and a return towards normal function of the liver following cessation of drug sue.

The effects of AS on the male reproductive system include: reductions in testosterone and gonadotropic hormones, sex hormone binding globulins; alterations in sperm number, motility and morphology; decreased testicular size, and abnormal appearance of testicular biopsy material. These effects have been shown in training studies (Clerico et al. 1981) studies of normal volunteers (Heller et al. 1959), therapeutic trials (Holma and Adlercreutz 1976), and studies of athletes self-administering AS (Alen and Suominen 1984; Hakkinen and Alen 1986; Ruokonen et al. 1985; Strauss et al. 1983). These changes have been shown to be reversible, but some of the effects may persist for months (Heller et al. 1959).

Other undesired effects of AS include their virilizing actions. These can be particularly problematic when they occur in young boys and women, both of whom are highly susceptible. AS have the capacity to cause premature epiphyseal closure, reducing ultimate height in children of both sexes. The masculinizing effects in females include deepening of the voice, clitoral enlargement, hirsutism, male pattern baldness, and reduction in breast size. Acne and alopecia may occur in both sexes, and males are also susceptible to gynecomastia as a result of AS use. AIDS has been reported in a bodybuilder, associated with the sharing of needles or injecting AS (Sklarek et al. 1984). AS may predispose athletes to connective tissue injuries (Wood et al. 1988). One case of prostate cancer in a bodybuilder has been reported recently (Roberts and Essenhigh 1986), and two bodybuilders have died from Wilms' tumor, at least one possibly associated with AS (Prat et al. 1977; Wright 1980). Although Kruskemper (1968) reports improved resistance with AS, one recent study found immunoglobins IgG, IgM, and IgA to be significantly lower in AS users than controls, suggesting the possibility of impaired humoral immunity associated with AS use (Calabrese et al. 1988).

Analysis of the adverse effects of androgens is complicated by various problems. Some effects are considered adverse only when they occur in inappropriate settings, such as the virilizing effects in women and children. Others result from the metabolites of the drugs, and since AS are metabolized differently, the side effects can vary equally. For example, some AS can be converted to estrogens and cause both virilizing and feminizing effects. Other adverse effects occur in response to drug actions that are unrelated to hormonal effects, such as the altered liver function caused by the 17-alpha alkyl (primarily oral) AS. Then, of course, there is considerable variability among individuals as to the incidence and severity of the various adverse effects.

In general, it is apparent that there is, indeed, a potential for long-term toxic effects. However, it has been stated that, in adult males at least, androgen abuse is probably not as dangerous as most other forms of drug abuse (Wilson 1988). Discontinuation of AS intake by males generally results in a cessation or reversal of virtually all virilizing and feminizing effects (Kruskemper 1968; Wilson 1988). Life threatening hepatic effects are extremely unusual, and the long-term consequences of blood lipid alterations are unclear. However, conventional wisdom and common sense suggest that these drugs are too powerful not to have some damaging effects with prolonged use. Furthermore, most use by athletes, and any possibly associated adverse effects, likely go undocumented and unreported. Unfortunately, the investigations necessary to assess the long-term health impact of the relatively well-studied short-term effects have not been performed. At present, therefore, despite the possible mitigating effects of intermittent use of these drugs and an otherwise healthy lifestyle, it would be imprudent to assume that athletes are immune from the deleterious effects observed in patients and animals.

In summary, AS are ergogenic when combined with the appropriate level of fitness, training volume and intensity, and nutritional program they are capable of facilitating increases in strength and lean body mass. However, they are also capable of inducing changes in various organs and body systems which are generally considered incompatible with optimal health, even if the users consider their subjective side effects insignificant.

Unfortunately few data are available on the incidence on prevalence of AS use. In the first national survey of AS use by high school students, nearly seven percent of male seniors admitted having used AS at least once (Buckley et al. 1988), and over one-third of those had used AS on five different occasions (cycles). These numbers probably represent a lower bound estimate. Use among elite athletes is certainly much higher (Yesalis et al. 1988) and likely much more prevalent in both sexes across the entire range of sports than has been believed.

The question of *why* is easily answered. We live in a highly competitive, chemically-oriented society that wants and expects instant gratification. The drugs have, in the past, been readily available. The non-medical use of AS has been estimated to be at least a $100-million-a-year *industry* in the United States. The episodes of drug use during the Olympics, as well as by college and professional athletes, seem not to be perceived by most athletes, recreational or competitive, as different from insider trading in the stock market, industrial espionage, scientists falsifying research, recruiting violations by coaches, or misconduct by students— they all seem to demonstrate that the end justifies the means. And, of course, use of AS is actually consistent with many of our societal values and behaviors. Bigger, taller, and leaner, more athletic, more assertive (aggressive) are better. Cosmetic medical intervention, from orthodontics to liposuction, breast augmentation (and reduction), hair transplantation, rhinoplasty, etc., with their attendant health risks, are increasingly commonplace.

Society has several options in dealing with misuse of AS. These include: investing more resources in: a) drug enforcement; b) drug testing; c) research and educational strategies; and d) reorienting our philosophy to focus more on the thrill of competition than on the thrill of victory.

Additional efforts in law enforcement, although appealing and definitely of some value, must be viewed realistically, given our seeming impotence in controlling the import, distribution, sale and use of other illicit drugs. Drug testing, particularly on a frequent, random, unannounced basis, would be extremely if not prohibitively expensive (at $100–200 per individual test) and may not stand up to the legal challenges it is sure to meet. Increased funding of research and more realistic educational strategies have a good deal of merit, especially since in some recent surveys 50 percent of users stated that they would seriously consider ceasing use if a significant incidence of truly deleterious health effects could be proven. However, even this approach would take many years, and a recent steroid education program in Oregon high schools had the effect of increasing rather than decreasing athletes' interests in using AS (Bosworth et al. 1988). Furthermore, if AS have been as widely and extensively used for many year as many believe, then why is there not more evidence on adverse health effects? The last option, reshaping our competitive nature and perspectives on athletics and physical culture, is likely to be as difficult as the others, particularly since so many facets of our culture and societal value systems are involved.

As Wilson (1988) has so aptly stated, this is one of those areas on the border between science and sociology. There are no easy answers, only difficult questions involving a potentially major public health problem. These can be effectively addressed only with a great deal of time, money, interest and commitment on the part of all persons with an interest in the values of physical activity to individual health and to society.

References

Alcena, V. and Alexopoulos, G. S. (1985) Ulcerative colitis in association with chronic paranoid schizophrenia: A review of steroid-induced psychiatric disorders. *Journal of Clinical Gastroenterology* 7:400–404.

Alen, M. (1985) Androgenic steroid effects on liver and red cells. *British Journal of Sports Medicine* 19:15–20.

Alen, M. and Suominen, J. (1984) Effect of androgenic and anabolic steroids on spermatogenesis in power athletes. *International Journal of Sports Medicine,* Supplement, 5:189–191.

American College of Sports Medicine (1984) Position stand on the use of anabolic-androgenic steroids in sports. *Sports Medicine Bulletin* 19:13–18.

Annitto, W. J. and Layman, W. A. (1980) Anabolic steroids and acute schizophrenic episode. *Journal of Clinical Psychiatry* 41:143–144.

Appell, H. J.; Heller-Umpfenbach, B.; Feraudi, M.; and Weicker, H. (1983) Ultrastructural and morphometric investigations on the effects of training and administration of anabolic steroids on the myocardium of guinea pigs. *International Journal of Sports Medicine* 4:268–274.

Arnold, A. P. (1984) Androgen regulation of motor neuron size and number. *Technology in Neural Sciences* 7:239–242.

Asano, A.; Wakasa, H.; Kaise, S.; Nishimaki, T.; and Kasukawa, R. (1982) Peliosis hepatis. Report on two autopsy cases with a review of literature. *Acta Pathologica Japanica* 32:861–877.

Bagheri, S. and Boyer, J. (1974) Peliosis hepatis associated with androgenic-anabolic steroid therapy—A severe form of hepatic injury. *Annals of Internal Medicine* 81:610–618.

Behrendt, H. (1977) Effect of anabolic steroids on rat heart muscle cells. I. Intermediate Filaments. *Cell Tissue Research* 180:303–315.

Behrendt, H. and Boffin, H. (1977) Myocardial cell lesions caused by an anabolic hormone. *Cell Tissue Research* 181:423–426.

Bosworth, E.; Bents, R.; Trevisan, L.; and Goldberg, L. (1988) Anabolic steroids and high school athletes. *Medicine and Science in Sports and Exercise* 20:53.

Buckley, W. E.; Yesalis, C. E., III; Friedl, K. E.; Anderson, W. A.; Streit, A. L.; and Wright, J. E. (1988) Estimated prevalence of anabolic steroid use among male high school seniors. *Journal of the American Medical Association* 260:3441–3445.

Byyny, R. L. (1976) Withdrawal from glucocorticoid therapy. *New England Journal of Medicine* 295:30–32.

Calabrese, L. H.; Kleiner, S.; Lombardo, J. (1987) The effects of anabolic steroids on the immune response in male body builders. *Medicine and Science in Sports and Exercise* 19:s52.

Clerico, A.; Ferdeghini, M.; and Palombo, C. (1981) Effects of anabolic treatment on the serum levels of gonadotropins, testosterone, prolactin, thyroid homrones and myoglobin of male athletes under physical training. *Journal of Nuclear Medicine and Allied Sciences* 25:79–88.

Cohen, J. C. and Hickman, R. (1987) Insulin resistance and diminished glucose tolerance in powerlifters ingesting anabolic steroids. *Journal of Clinical Endocrinology and Metabolism* 65:960–963.

Dahlmann, B.; Widjaja, A.; and Reinauer, H. (1981) Antagonistic effects of endurance training and testosterone on alkaline proteolytic activity in rat skeletal muscle. *European Journal of Applied Physiology* 46:229–235.

Dequeker, J. and Geusens, P. (1985) Anabolic steroids and osteoporosis. *Acta Endocrinologica* 271:45–52.

Freinhar, J. P. and Alvarez, W. (1985) Androgen-induced hypomania. Letter to the Editor. *Journal of Clinical Psychiatry* 46:354–355.

Goodman, L. S. and Gilman, A. (Eds.) (1975) *The Pharmacological Basis of Therapeutics.* New York: Macmillan.

Hakkinen, K. and Alen, M. (1986) Physiological performance, serum hormones, enzymes and lipids of an elite power athlete during training with and without androgens and during prolonged detraining. A case study. *Journal of Sports Medicine and Physical Fitness* 26:92–100.

Haupt, H. A. and Rovere, G. D. (1984) Anabolic steroids: A review of the literature. *American Journal of Sports Medicine* 12:469–484.

Heller, C. G.; Moore, D. J.; Paulsen, C. A.; Nelson, W. O.; and Laidlaw, W. M. (1959) Effects of progesterone and synthetic progestins on the reproductive physiology of normal men. *Federation Proceedings* 18:1057–1065.

Hervey, G. R.; Hutchinson, I.; Knibbs, A. V.; Burkinshaw, L.; Jons, P. R. M.; Noland, N. G.; and Levell, M. J.(1976) "Anabolic" effects of methadienone in men undergoing athletic training. *Lancet* 2:699–702.

Hervey, G. R.; Knibbs, A. V.; Burkinshaw, L.; Morgan, D. B.; Jones, P. R. M.; Chettle, D. R.; and Vartsky, D. (1981) Effects of methadienone on the performance and body composition of men undergoing athletic training. *Clinical Science* 60:457–461.

Hickson, R. C.; Galassi, T. M.; Kurowski, T. T.; Daniels, D. G.; and Chatterton, R. T., Jr. (1983) Skeletal muscle cytosol (3H)methyl trienolone receptor binding and serum androgens: Effects of hypertrophy and hormonal state. *Journal of Steroid Biochemistry* 19:1705.

Holma, P. and Adlercreutz, H. (1976) Effects of an anabolic steroid (Methadienone) on plasma LH-FSH and testosterone and on the response to intravenous administration of LHRH. *Acta Endocrinologica* 83:856–864.

Holma. P. (1977) Effect of an anabolic steroid (Methadienone) on central and peripheral blood flow in well trained male athletes. *Annals of Clinical Research* 9:215–221.

Hurley, B. F.; Seas, D. R.; Hagberg, J. M.; Goldberg, A. C.; Ostrove, S. M.; Holloszy, J. O.; Weist, W. G.; and Goldberg, A. P. (1984) High density-lipoprotein cholesterol in bodybuilders and powerlifters (negative effects of androgens). *Journal of the American Medical Association* 252:507–513.

Ishak, K. G. (1981) Hepatic lesions caused by anabolic and contraceptive steroids. *Seminars in Liver Disease* 1:116–128.

Itil, T. M.; Cora, R.; Akpinar, S.; Herrmann, W. M.; and Patterson, C. J. (1974) "Psychotropic" action of sex hormones: Computerized EEG in establishing the immediate CNS effects of steroid hormones. *Current Therapeutic Research* 16:1147–1170.

Itil, T. M. (1976)Neurophysiological effects of hormones in humans: Computer EEG profiles of sex and hypothalamic hormones. In E.J. Sachar (Ed.) *Hormones, Behavior and Psychotherapy.* New York: Raven Press.

Kochakian, C. D. (Ed.) (1976) *Anabolic-Androgenic Steroids.*New York: Springer-Verlag.

Kopera, H. (1985) The history of anabolic steroid and a review of clinical experience with anabolic steroids. *Acta Endocrinologica* 110:11–18.

Kruskemper, H. L. (1968) *Anabolic Steroids.* New York: Academic Press.

Kurz, E. M.; Sengelaub, D. R.; and Arnold, A. P. (1986) Androgens regulate the dendrite length of mammalian motorneurons in adulthood. *Science* 232: 395–398.

Lamb, D. R. (1984) Anabolic steroids sin athletics: How well do they work and how dangerous are they? *The American Journal of Sports Medicine* 12:31–38.

Lewis, D. A. and Smith, R. E. (1983) Steroid-induced psychiatric syndromes. *Journal of Affective Disorders* 5:319–332.

Morano, I. (1984) Influence of exercise and dianabol on the degradation rate of myofibrillar proteins of the heart and three fiber types of skeletal muscle of female guinea pigs. *International Journal of Sports Medicine* 5:317.

Nagelberg, S. B.; Laue, L.; Loriaux, D. L.; Liu, L.; and Sherins, R. J. (1986) Cerebrovascular accident associated with testosterone therapy in a 21-year-old hypogonadal male. *New England Journal of Medicine* 314:649–650.

National Strength and Conditioning Association (1985) Position paper on anabolic drug use by athletes. *National Strength and Conditioning Association,* Lincoln, NE.

Olsson, A. G.; Oro, L.; and Rossner, S. (1974) Effects of oxandrolone on plasma lipoproteins and the intravenous fat tolerance in man. *Atherosclerosis* 19:337–346.

Orlandi, F. and Jezequel, A. M. (1972) *Liver and Drugs.* New York: Academic Press.

O'Shea, J. P. (1978) Anabolic steroids in sport: A biophysiological evaluation. *Nutrition Reports International* 17:607–627.

Overly, W. L.; Dankoff, J. A.; Wang, B. K.; and Singh, U. D. (1984) Androgens and hepatocellular carcinoma in an athlete. *Annals of Internal Medicine* 100: 158–159.

Paradinas, F. J.; Bull, T. B.; Westaby, D.; and Murray-Lyon, I. M. (1977) Hyperplasia and prolapse of hepatocytes into hepatic veins during long-term methyl testosterone therapy: Possible relations;hips of these changes to the development of peliosis hepatis and liver tumors. *Histopathology* 1:225–246.

Peters, J. H.; Randall, A. H.; Mendeloff, J.; Peace, R.; Coberly, J. C.; and Hurley, M. B. (1958) Jaundice during administration of methylestrenolone. *Journal of Clinical Endocrinology* 18:114–115.

Pope, H. G. and Katz, D. L. (1988) Affective and psychotic symptoms associated with anabolic steroid use. *American Journal of Psychiatry* 145:487–490.

Prat, J.; Gray, G. F.; Stolley, P. D.; and Coleman, J. W. (1977) Wilms' tumor in an adult associated with androgen abuse. *Journal of the American Medical Association* 21:2322–2323.

Puffer, J. C. (1986) The use of drugs in swimming. *Clinics in Sports Medicine* 5:77.

Rance, N. E. and Max, S. R. (1984) Modulation of the cytosolic androgen receptor in striated muscle by sex steroids. *Endocrinology* 115:862–866.

Roberts, J. T. and Essenhigh, D. M. (1986) Adenocarcinoma of prostate in 40-year-old bodybuilder. *Lancet* 2:742.

Ruokonen, A.; Alen, M.; Bolton, N.; and Vihko, R. (1985) Response of serum testosterone and its precursor steroids, SHBG and CBG to anabolic steroid and testosterone self-administration in men. *Journal of Steroid Biochemistry* 23:33–38.

Ryan, A. J. (1976) Athletics. In C. D. Kochakian (Ed.) *Anabolic-Androgenic Steroids.* Springer-Verlag, New York.

Salgado, E. and Selye, H. (1954) The production of hypertension, nephrosclerosis and cardiac lesions by methyl-androstenediol treatment in the rat. *Endocrinology* 55:550–560.

Sar, M. and Stumpf, W. E. (1977) Androgen concentration in motor neurons of cranial nerves and spinal cord. *Science* 197:77–79.

Schaffner, F.; Popper, H.; and Chesrow, E. (1959) Cholestasis produced by the administration of norethandrolone. *American Journal of Medicine* 26:249–254.

Schaffner, F.; Popper, H.; and Perez, V. (1960) Changes in bile canaliculi produced by norethandrolone: Electron microscopic study of human and rat liver. *Journal of Laboratory and Clinical Medicine* 56:623–628.

Sherlock, S. (1979) Effects of androgens and contraceptive steroids on liver function in humans. *Advances in Pharmacy and Therapeutics* 8:149–158.

Shiozawa, Z.; Yamada, H.; Mabuchi, C.; Hotta, T.; Saito, M.; Sabue, I.; and Huang, W. P. (1982)Superior sagittal sinus thrombosis associated with androgen therapy for hypoplastic anemia. *Annals of Neutology* 12:578–580.

Sklarek, H. M.; Mantovani, R. P.; Erens, E.; Heiler, D.; Niederman, M. S.; and Fein, A. M. (1984) AIDS in a bodybuilder using anabolic steroids. *New England Journal of Medicine* 311:1701.

Stang-Voss, C. and Appell, H. J. (1981) Structural alterations of liver parenchyma induced by anabolic steroids. *International Journal of Sports Medicine* 2:101–105.

Strauss, R. H.; Wright, J. E.; Finerman, G. A. M.; and Catlin, D. H. (1983) Side effects of anabolic steroids in weight-trained men. *Physician and Sports Medicine* 11:87–96.

Stromme, S. B.; Meen, H. D.; And Aakvaag, A. (1974) Effects of an androgenic-anabolic steroid on strength development and plasma testosterone levels in normal males. *Medicine and Science in Sports* 6:203–208.

Stumpf, W. E. and Sar, M. (1976) Steroid hormone target sites in the brain: The differential distribution of estrogen, progestin, androgen and glucocorticosteroid. *Journal of Steroid Biochemistry* 7:1163–1170.

Taylor, W.; Snowball, S.; Dickerson, C. M.; and Lesna, M. (1982) Alterations of liver architecture in mice treated with anabolic androgens and diethynitrosamine. *NATO Advanced Study Institute Series,* SEries A. 52:279–288.

Tennant, F.; Black, D. L.; and Voy, R. O. (1988) Anabolic steroid dependence with opioid-type features. *New England Journal of Medicine* 319:579.

Turner, R. (1981) The value of anabolic steroids for patients receiving chemotherapy. *Clinical Oncology Society,* Australia Annual Meeting, APCS, No. 9. Found in *Excerpta Medica:* Princeton, Geneva, Amsterdam.

Venable, J. H. (1966) Morphology of the cells of normal, testosterone-deprived and testosterone-stimulated levator ani muscles. *American Journal of Anatomy* 119:271.

Vyskocil, F. and Gutmann, E. (1977)Electropysioilogical and contractile properties of the levator ani muscle after castration and testosterone administration. *Pflugers Archives* 368:104–109.;

Webb, O. L.; Laskarzewski, P. M.; and Glueck, C. J. (1984) Severe depression of high-density lipoprotein cholesterol levels in weightlifters and bodybuilders by self-administered exogenous testosterone and anabolic-androgenic steroids. *Metabolism* 33:971–975.

Williams, M. H. (1974) *Drugs and Athletic Performance.* Springfield, IL: Thomas.

Wilson, J. D. (1988) *t*Androgen abuse by athletes. *Endocrine Reviews* 9:181–199.

Wilson, J. D. and Gloyna, E. (1970) The intranuclear metabolism of testosterone in the accessory organs of male reproduction. *Recent Progress in Hormone Research* 26:309.

Wilson, J. D. and Griffin, J. E. (1980) The use and misuse of androgens. *Metabolism* 29:1278–1295.

Wood, T. O.; Cooke, P. H.; and Goodship, A. E. (1988) The effect of exercise and anabolic steroids on the mechanical properties and crimp morphology of the rat tendon. *American Journal of Sports Medicine* 16:153–158.

Wright, J. E. (1978) *Anabolic Steroids and Sports.* Natick, MA: Sports Science Consultants.

Wright, J. E. (1980) Anabolic steroids and athletics. In R. S Hutton and D. I. Muller (Eds.) *Exercise and Sports Science Reviews* 8:149–202.

Wright, J. E. (1982) *Anabolic Steroids and Sports.* Volume II. Natick, MA: Sports Science Consultants.

Yesalis, C.; Herrick, R.; Buckley, W.; Friedl, K.; Brannon, D.; and Wright, J. (1988) Estimated incidence of anabolic steroid use among elite powerlifters. *Physician and Sports Medicine* 16:91–100.

CHAPTER 5

PSYCHOLOGICAL FACTORS IN THE USE OF RECREATIONAL DRUGS AND ALCOHOL

Steven R. Heyman, Ph.D.

Overview

This chapter is designed to examine the key psychological factors relating to athletes' use and abuse of recreational drugs and alcohol. While it is assumed that athletes are vulnerable to the same range of factors that cause recreational substance use and abuse in the general society, there are factors that can take on particular significance for athletes. After reviewing a series of these key factors, the implications of these factors for the athlete and the sport world will be discussed.

Most of the comparisons between athlete and nonathlete use of alcohol and drugs suggest little overall differences (Bell and Doege 1987; Clement 1983; Duda 1986). There are some specific differences that may be important and will be discussed later. At the same time, this lack of overall difference should not obscure an important assumption. It is generally conceded there are a variety of different reasons for drug and alcohol use (Sarason and Sarason 1984). It is an important assumption of this chapter that certain reasons are likely to be more relevant to athletes. Naturally, to understand a specific individual's usage pattern would require an understanding of that individual. Specific factors, or combinations of factors, will be differentially relevant to varied individuals.

"Recreational Drugs" and "Recreational Use": Confusing Terms

In writing this chapter there were several difficult beginning points due to our society's ambivalent attitudes toward alcohol and drug use. The concept of a *recreational drug* implies an illegal drug, such as cocaine, that can be used by some for pleasure on an intermittent basis. At the same time, however, individuals can be arrested for the possession or distribution of these substances. A great deal of money is also spent to discourage the use of these drugs.

If there is a lack of clarity around the term recreational drugs, there is also uncertainty around the concept of *recreational use.* This implies that drugs or alcohol can be used occasionally, for pleasure or for fun, without being detrimental to the individual or to society. There is a general recognition of this for alcohol. Again, most recreational drugs are outlawed, but there is an implicit assumption, particularly among certain subgroups, that these substances can be used occasionally, for recreation. Still, considerable amounts of time and money are expended to prevent the use of these substances. Perhaps the best known of these campaigns is the "Just Say No" program.

This chapter cannot attempt to resolve this confusion. There are also fads in drug use (Ryan 1984). A decade ago, LSD might have been used widely enough for it to be considered in this recreational category more prominently than it will be in this chapter. In another decade different drugs might be considered. In this chapter, drugs such as heroin, crack, and freebase are not considered recreational drugs; both because of their less common use in general and by athletes, and because of the general recognition of their dangerous and addictive qualities. Cocaine, marijuana, amphetamines, and barbiturates will be principally considered in addition to alcohol.

Where appropriate, there will be differentiations made between the recreational use of drugs and alcohol, and substance abuse. This is not an easy differentiation to make. There are individuals who will experiment with a drug or alcohol, perhaps using the substance for a few times, and then never again. Others may use drugs or alcohol on an occasional basis, but an overall view of their usage patterns would suggest a pattern controlled both in frequency and quantity. This pattern would generally qualify as recreational. The last major term, abuse, is more difficult to determine. It is not easy to state how frequent a use, in what quantities, or what combination of frequency and use, will constitute abuse. This chapter will try to recognize and deal with some of the differences between recreational use and abuse as they relate to athletes.

Biopsychological Factors and Athlete Recreational Drug Use

Sensation Seeking, Augmenting-Reducing, and Related Concepts

Although drugs can be classified in a number of ways, there are two broad categories: stimulants and depressants. Some drugs fit fairly clearly into one or the other category: barbiturates are depressants, and amphetamines and cocaine are stimulants. Although alcohol is a central nervous system depressant, it has a mixed effect on individuals, depending on quantity, personal factors, etc. Due likely to its ability to release inhibitions and its initial effects on blood circulation, alcohol can appear to act as a stimulant. Marijuana does not fit well into either category.

Zuckerman (1979) has published a variety of studies on what he has called *sensation seeking*. Some individuals have a particularly greater ability to tolerate higher levels of sensory and neurological stimulation. In fact, these individuals are likely to seek out such stimulations. There has not been a systematic study of athletes by sport and sensation seeking, but several studies have shown high risk sport athletes, in particular, to be more sensation seeking (Heyman and Rose 1980; 1981; Straub 1982).

Zuckerman's findings, and those of others dealing with related concepts such as *augmenting and reducing* (Petrie 1967) and strength of the nervous system (Sales et al. 1971), suggest neurobiological differences between individuals that may well predispose them to different types of behaviors.

Relative to drugs, although research findings have not always been consistent, Zuckerman has reported that higher sensation seekers are more likely to use stimulants, while lower sensation seekers are more likely to select depressants. Alcohol and marijuana did not have clear relationships to personality types, likely due to their mixed psychological and pharmacological actions. It is worthwhile noting Toohey (1978) found few differences between athletes and nonathletes in drug usage at five universities; but at one university athletes were more likely to use amphetamines, while at four universities they were less likely to use barbiturates.

Not all athletes will be sensation seekers. Certain sports, however, requiring high levels of stimulation, sensory input, and response, may be more likely to attract higher sensation seekers. Such individuals would be likely to be more successful in such situations.

It may not be a coincidence that cocaine appears to have become so prominent in athletic circles. It seems likely that within athletes as a group, and perhaps particularly in such sports as football, basketball, hockey, and boxing, there may be a greater number of high sensation seekers, individuals who neurobiologically are programmed to want, to tolerate, and to enjoy higher levels of sensory stimulation, such as can be achieved by using cocaine and other stimulants.

Having found these levels of stimulation available through drugs, it may be more difficult to abandon the immediacy and intensity of these experiences. While cocaine may not be physically addictive, it may be a particular danger for those who want and can tolerate greater levels of stimulation. Not only may cocaine fulfill these needs, but as with any stimulant, it will create feelings of satisfaction, well-being, power, and even omnipotence, depending on the individual and the dosage. Smith (1983) has discussed the addiction to sensation and experience, alcohol problem predispositions, and the athlete environment.

The causes of alcohol abuse are not clearly understood and are certainly widely debated and controversial. Evidence does suggest that certain individuals have an inherited predisposition to alcohol abuse (Sarason and Sarason 1984). As a basic statement, individuals born to alcoholic parents, but raised from birth by nonalcoholic adoptive parents, still have a higher risk for alcohol-related problems than does the general population.

There is no evidence to indicate that athletes, either by sport or as a group, have a greater inherited tendency towards alcohol abuse. However, for the individuals with such a predisposition, being placed in an environment that encourages drinking, and particularly frequent and heavy drinking, may trigger the problem situation. Although this will be discussed in more detail later in this chapter, the athletic environment often encourages frequent and heavy drinking, and can create the worst environment for athletes who come to it with a predisposition for abuse.

Contributing Factors in the Sport World

Did the Sport World Open the Door?

Social learning theory, particularly the work of Bandura and Walters (1963), has helped us to understand much about how people learn their social behaviors, and the situations under which they express these behaviors.

We might think that the sport environment, with its emphasis on health, would present an ideal environment militating against the abuse of alcohol as well as the use and abuse of recreational drugs. Perhaps for a long time these behaviors were inhibited in athletes due to positive factors in the sport environment and peer relationships.

Unfortunately, other factors have come into play over the last two decades. Certainly the sport environment has never actively encouraged the abuse of alcohol or recreational drugs. Our society, in general, has become highly drug oriented. Edwards (1987) estimates that by the time an individual is twenty-one, he or she will have seen approximately 150,000 commercials for legally available drugs, guaranteed to provide rapid solutions for a variety of problems. One also quickly learns that even more potent drugs are available only by prescription. These affect all segments of society, not just athletes. Even in the face of social factors and a youth subculture that has become oriented towards recreational drugs, environments like the sporting world, stressing healthier lifestyles, should influence against alcohol and drug abuse.

Unfortunately, over the last decades, the sport environment, through modeling and disinhibition, has opened the door to alcohol and recreational drug use, even if unknowingly. Modeling suggests that we are more likely to imitate the behaviors of individuals we see as important, attractive, powerful, etc. Disinhibition indicates that certain conditions will facilitate the expression of behaviors previously held in check.

Due to the pressures of competition, beginning in the 1950's, the sporting environment began relying on drugs to facilitate athlete performance. Amphetamines were used by players to enhance performance and alter mood. Other drugs could be used to reduce pain and swelling, to allow for continued participation. Steroids were actively encouraged to facilitate muscle growth and strength, as well as to enhance competitive mood.

The intent of the sporting environment relative to these drugs was, no doubt, specific to competition. The encouragement to use drugs, however, to perform and to feel better, also suggests more broadly that the use of drugs is acceptable. Vulnerable individuals, in an environment that did not encourage drug use, might have stayed away from such usage. The encouragement to use drugs by significant individuals may well have weakened their safeguards and disinhibited their controls.

By opening the door to the use of drugs, the sport environment could not have anticipated the results. Through modeling and disinhibition a sense of permission was given, and this synchronized with an era in which recreational drug use became common. These factors made it easier for athletes to move from specific types of drugs to greater use of alcohol and recreational drugs, particularly as peers engaged in these behaviors.

It is proving far more difficult to close this door, in part because segments of the sport environment have not taken a uniform stand on drug use. As the sport sociologist Harry Edwards (1987, p. 3) has said,

> "... to educate about one category of abused drugs without focusing upon the other with equal urgency would be to perpetrate an existing hypocrisy and to exacerbate rather than ameliorate the confusion and contradictions surrounding the drug problems in sports."

Ryan (1984) also voices similar opinions.

The Male Role Macho: Implications for Athlete Alcohol and Drug Use

Modeling, unfortunately, has also had its effects in other ways. To a great extent in our society, alcohol use has been tied to the male sex role: macho men can drink a great deal, and often. In general, athletes of both sexes are likely to be considerably more masculine (even as part of androgyny) in their sex role orientation (Ugoccioni and Ballantyne 1980). While this will allow them to be more aggressive and competitive in sport situations, they may be more vulnerable to the negative expressions of this sex role orientation in other settings. To prove how tough they are, athletes may therefore be even more vulnerable to alcohol and drug use than might other groups.

Alcohol abuse by sport celebrities is not new—the press has simply been more open about reporting it. Until recently, however, this use, and abuse, has not been consistently presented in a negative light. One great football star, when asked what he did to prepare the night before a winning Super Bowl performance, is reported to have said, "Got a bottle of booze and a broad." Certainly macho. The effects on younger athletes in particular, can be very negative.

In reviewing advertisements for certain types of alcoholic beverages, particularly for beer (which can be advertised on television, unlike hard liquor), we find a high percentage of athletes. A Special Report (1982) stated that 90% of the spokesmen for a major light beer were athletes. Similarly, we find beer manufacturers are among the major sponsors of sporting events. The Special Report (1982) found that one of every 4.2 commercials televised during network sports was for beer. The message is quite clear: if you are an athlete, you can, and should, drink beer, often.

The athletic system makes it clear at sporting events alcohol should be consumed. What child, going to baseball, football, boxing, hockey, basketball, etc., will not see a number of the spectators drinking beer, and often in great quantities? This again is likely to have a profound impact, and the behaviors observed can be easily expressed later, particularly if the sport environment continues to give mixed messages about alcohol and drug use.

Due to the association of alcohol use and masculinity in our culture, athletes, both male and female, may be more vulnerable to abuse than might other groups. We no longer live in a culture, however, of simple alcohol abuse. As J. Pursch, M.D. notes, "You rarely see a pure alcoholic anymore . . . if they're under 40, they're chemical gourmets" (Special Report 1982, p. 116).

Finally, in our society we generally use alcohol to celebrate victories and to drown sorrows. The athletic environment has not said to this tradition "no, not here." In fact, the opposite appears to have been the case. How often in locker rooms, after a victory, do we see athletes gulping from bottles of champagne? How often, in interviews with winners and losers, do athletes talk about going out, implying or stating they will get drunk? Unfortunately—all too often—and this sets a model for younger athletes.

Again, the sport world certainly did not create the association between alcohol (or drugs) and celebration or mourning. With the relationship between masculine sex role behaviors and sport, the increased use and abuse of alcohol and drugs becomes possible for participants, particularly as admired athletes model these behaviors.

Peer Influences

It is generally assumed that peer values affect drug use, particularly among adolescents. It seems reasonable, though, that individuals likely to use recreational drugs will affiliate with other similar individuals, and perhaps only in a smaller number of cases are individuals pressured to engage in behaviors they find unacceptable. An individuals's self-esteem, identity, and social skills would contribute to a decision and an ability to resist drug or alcohol use, or to change peer groups.

It may be easier for a person who finds a peer group developing disliked behaviors, like alcohol and drug use, to change groups of friends than it is for an athlete to change teams or teammates. Although large teams may have subgroups with different behaviors, this may be less likely on smaller teams.

At the same time, athletes are often taught to think and work together. Therefore, one group, pressing alcohol or drug use, may gain considerable influence over other individuals, particularly those who are uncertain or neutral in their attitudes towards alcohol and drug use. Even when an individual or subgroup might want actively to oppose alcohol or drug use, for the sake of team harmony, cohesiveness, the upcoming games, etc., their views may be moderated.

Where team members have truly learned to believe "there is no I in team," it may be more difficult to resist the pressures or invitations of others. As individual members become more oriented toward alcohol or drugs, either because of their enthusiasm about their new experiences, or because of their own uncertainties, they may overstate the positiveness of these experiences. Not only may their descriptions sound attractive, but the experience of peer pressure will be coupled with a norm that the group members should be alike. With too great a stress on thinking and acting alike, on submerging one's individuality, the less confident and perhaps younger individuals may be at greater risk for conforming to the alcohol and drug use patterns.

We might assume that an athlete would have boundaries between team conformity relating to the sport, and conformity outside the sport. Unfortunately, this may be less the case than would be desired. Particularly in smaller schools, athletes may have their primary friendships and identifications around the team. They spend a great deal of time together, dress alike, talk alike, and think alike.

Even where this press to conformity may be less, or may not exist, athletes are often required to spend a great deal of time together: practices, competitions, road trips, etc. It may be considerably more difficult to resist the temptation to become involved with teammates and friends under these conditions of close association.

If the group values are positive and prevent alcohol or drug use, this may be seen as a desirable condition. As an individual, or groups of individuals, begin to express other behaviors, the press to conformity may come to work against the positive values. The individuals who begin the use of alcohol or drugs may be less conforming than others and have a greater motivation to change their peers' values.

Masculinity, the Male Sex Role, and Athlete Alcohol and Drug Use

Within our society, alcohol usage and abuse rates have traditionally been higher for males than for females. No clear comparisons exist for athletes, as a group or by sport, as compared with nonathletes. Particularly for adolescent males, however, there has been as association of alcohol use and toughness, with an emphasis on periods of heavy and frequent alcohol use. Where frequency and amount of use becomes the test, recreational drugs can substitute for, or be used along with, alcohol.

Athletes may be more vulnerable to such use and abuse because of the hypermasculine environment in which they function. Mixed sex groups may dampen the aggressive and competitive patterns more likely to be found in all male groups. Male athletes, spending a great deal of time together in practice, on the road and after games, may well be more vulnerable to the use of alcohol and drugs as measures of toughness.

We might assume the reverse would be true for female athletes. Unfortunately, just as the equalization of male and female roles in society has been accompanied with higher rates of alcohol and substance abuse problems for women, this also seems to be the case for female athletes. Duda (1986, p. 146) reports that studies have found little differences between male and female athletes drug usage patterns. In fact, a slightly greater percentage of female athletes reported regular use of alcohol. Duda comments, "Celebrating victories and drowning sorrows has long been a tradition associated with sport, and female athletes have joined in." Similarly, Saunders reported nearly one in four Big 10 women's coaches have reported that their teams were involved in excessive social use of alcohol, and 14% of high school coaches had helped their female athletes seek professional help for drinking problems (Special Report 1982).

"Drug use by women will follow the same pattern as for men. . . .
They are using cocaine to be up for games, and are having to cope
with the emotional plummet that follows. They are using marijuana
[in the same ways as the men do]" (p. 118).

At the same time, as was noted previously, female athletes are more
likely to have a masculine or an androgynous sex role orientation. They
are also placed in an environment that has been heavily oriented to male
values and behaviors, whereas until recently, they have often been
"second class citizens." They may model the male behaviors due to a
combination of these factors, including the usage of alcohol and recreational drugs.

Athletes, Stress, and Stress Reduction: The Role of Alcohol and Recreational Drugs

To a great extent, many individuals who use or abuse alcohol and
drugs will give stress reduction as a reason. Athletes face unique stressors, often to greater extent than their nonathlete counterparts.

In school, at all levels, athletes are typically required to complete
the same coursework as nonathletes, but are also required to spend additional time in practice and competition. Some can handle both sets of re-
quirements nicely, and can deal with the typical developmental issues
confronting them. Others will find meeting the demands of all of these
situations considerably more stressful.

As athletes get older, their peers may be concentrating on careers
and families, usually with time schedules that are reasonably compatible,
while athletes may find schedules in conflict with each other. The hours
of practice, competition, and travel, may well interfere with one's personal life, and all too often, athletes postpone career considerations until
after the athletic career is ended.

Not unrelated, competitive athletes are aware that their careers will
eventually end: few will go on to college teams, even fewer will go on to
professional sports. Elite athletes are aware that each year younger athletes are waiting to replace them.

For both younger and more mature athletes, the constancy of practice, road trips, and preparing for peak performance in competition adds
to the stress they experience. Quite often athletes, and the pressures they
experience, may not be understood by nonathletes (Nicholi 1983), adding
to the sense of isolation and loneliness that they may have.

Some athletes, as they experience the stressors they encounter, may find feelings of anxiety. Others, as the result of physical and/or psychological exhaustion, may experience depression. There are medically prescribed drugs for both of these, however to admit to these feelings would be to admit to having problems. Taking recreational drugs may alleviate these feelings, but because of the social situation the presence of problems can be denied.

Perhaps particularly during long and boring road trips, or periods away from home, family, and friends—but at other times as well—the ready availability of drugs and alcohol may increase the likelihood for their usage. Unfortunately, as a society we have become oriented to chemical means of stress reduction.

As the sport world became more oriented to the use of chemicals to enhance performance, it may have opened the door for athletes to use alcohol and drugs to reduce stress. While the occasional use of alcohol or certain drugs for recreation might not be a serious issue, the use of these substances for stress reduction can become quite problematic. As long as the stressors persist, a person, through basic conditioning, may associate relief with alcohol and drugs and become dependent on these substances. It is also impossible to predict who is more prone to developing abuse problems once usage begins. Certainly not all will—but definitely some will.

Not only may alcohol or drugs be used to reduce the feelings of stress, they can also be used to avoid the recognition of stressful situations. It is this writer's clinical observation, and it is shared by others, that athletes, as they face career termination, or disruptions due to accident, injury, or replacement, are more prone to increasing rates of alcohol and recreational drugs usage. This seems, in part, to lower the stress, but it also is to avoid dealing with the reality of the situation.

For some the extent of the stress may require not only an excessive amount of alcohol or drug for temporary relief, but the psychological and physical relief may only come after the exhaustion of excess. One athlete seen in therapy by this writer, for example, would expend considerable energy in mental and physical preparation for competition. When the competition was over, however, he found himself unable to relax. Considerable amounts of alcohol and cocaine were consumed, not only for immediate gratification, but for the purposes of inducing an exhaustion, and only that brought a great sense of relief. Considerable therapeutic work was required to understand the situation and develop more positive personal patterns.

Personal Factors in Athlete Alcohol and Drug Use

Negative Identities

Dumb Jock

Within our society we often express admiration and even idolize athletes. Like so many things, however, there is also a negative side to the athlete identity. The psychoanalyst Erik Erikson (1968), in discussing the development of identity, dealt with negative identities: ones which are not acceptable to most of society, but which help an individual form a bond with others perceived as similar, to relieve feelings of alienation, isolation, etc. Usually when we think of such individuals or groups, we might think of the Hell's Angels, or perhaps Punk Rockers.

It is understood that the term *dumb jock* may be offensive to some. To understand the negative identity, it must be used. The power of the term is important in understanding its impact on the athlete.

We too often have the stereotype of the dumb jock. While we idolize athletes for skill and prowess, we demean their intellectual abilities. It can become easy for an individual who has heard this often enough to believe it, or to seek actively to dissociate themselves from it.

In a number of cases, particularly at the high school and college levels, athletes who may not have been oriented toward alcohol or drug usage, may find peers using these substances. Their unwillingness to use alcohol or drugs may not be seen by others as a personal or health decision, but as a manifestation of being a dumb jock.

Psychology tells us in such situations an individual's values may be in conflict. They will experience cognitive dissonance, which carries a form of anxiety with it. To eliminate this conflict, values and/or behaviors must change. The basic choices in the situation cited above would be to view the friends less positively and to hold to one's views against alcohol or drug use, or to change one's attitudes and behaviors relative to alcohol and drug use, and continue the relationships.

Similar patterns may await older athletes, particularly at the professional level. In the late 1970's and early 1980's cocaine use soared among college students, as well as among celebrities in society. Athletes were sought out by celebrities and were likely exposed to ready access to this drug, as well as to others. An athlete who comes from a different social class, or who has been used to associating with more conventional individuals, may again feel like an outsider, perhaps a dumb jock. To relieve these feelings it may have been easier to do what the popular and attractive group was doing.

It has not been uncommon for athletes who have developed substance abuse problems to discuss the readiness of individuals to provide them with drugs, with as cocaine, in return for allowing these individuals to associate with them. Edwards (1987) states that 80% of athletes get their drugs from friends or relatives: few need to use unknown dealers.

Perhaps with a better sense of self and self-worth, athletes would be less vulnerable to alcohol and drug use and abuse.

Rebellion

We assume, as part of adolescence, all adolescents develop a sense of self, to a degree, by asserting themselves against parental or societal values. Athletes, both younger and older, can live in a tightly controlled world in which many of their patterns are dictated to them: where to live, to eat, when to work or go to school, when to practice, when to be in, etc. Athletes can become part of an overall public relations program, in which appearances are more important than reality. It has been an unfortunate observation by a number of athletes, for example, that many sport programs are less concerned about athlete drug use because of its effects on athletes, and more concerned about its effect on public relations.

In such a system, the use of alcohol, and perhaps particularly recreational drugs, can provide an athlete with a sense of covertly rebelling against authority, against the system, or other forces beyond his or her control: and at the same time, a rebellion that is physically pleasurable. For the athlete, this rebellion would have the particular benefit of secretly belying the publicly erected image, giving the individual an enhanced inner sense of victory.

Aggression

We place athletes in a particularly difficult situation regarding the expression of aggressive feelings. We encourage athletes, particularly in contact sports, but also in *noncontact* sports such as basketball, to be physically aggressive in the competitive situation. We also maintain that this behavior should not be expressed in nonsport situations. Most athletes do not have difficulties with this. For some however, this separation is more difficult to make. By encouraging the expression of these behaviors in the sport situation, we may make it more difficult for some to control these feelings in other situations.

Alcohol and drug use for some athletes may be the vehicle by which the expression of these feelings is legitimized: "I wouldn't have done that if I hadn't been drunk/stoned/high/coked-up." For others, the more tenuous controls on these patterns may truly be loosened by the alcohol or drug experience. Where alcohol or drug use is associated with toughness, the interaction of these factors with aggression can be very problematic. Too often has this writer heard of teams who go out with the intent of getting high and looking for fights. In two cases, individuals with particular problems in these areas have been referred, one by a court and one by a coach. Alcohol and drugs are also likely to contribute to feelings of power and strength that can also combine with aggressive attitudes.

The sporting environment has not consistently addressed the needs to keep physically aggressive feelings in check out of the sport situation. To some extent, the expression of these behaviors has been reinforced by peers, who might want to see a good fight, and by officials, who have assumed it is more acceptable for athletes to engage in such behaviors. In some cases, athletes have been protected by school or law enforcement officials because of their status or value to a team. Unfortunately, the role of alcohol and drugs in these situations has been minimized or not dealt with.

"I Could've Been a Contender"

Athletes, like other individuals, are confronted both by their potential and by the public demonstration of their abilities. For those who are unsure of themselves, or for those who do not have the abilities expected by others, alcohol and drug use becomes a convenient way to minimize performance. That is, an athlete may be able to say, "Imagine what I could have done if I hadn't been so high!"

Sadly, there may also be a peer reinforcement for this. An athlete, even with lowered performance due to his or her alcohol or drug usage, may be seen as accomplishing greater feats by a subgroup oriented toward alcohol or drug use.

Mood Alteration

Although other chapters in this volume will deal with the ergogenic aspects of drugs, it is important to note that athletes may use drugs or alcohol, not only for perceived physical advantages, but for psychological arousal and motivation, as well as for mood alteration (Mandell et al. 1981; Ryan 1984).

Stimulants in particular, such as amphetamines or cocaine, can elevate mood and enhance feelings of confidence. These can be utilized when physical or psychological exertion has become extreme, and the individual's personal resources are experienced as exhausted. At the same time, athletes in conflict may also use these to reduce the feelings of conflict and to enhance the sense of well-being. For example, one athlete felt considerable pressure by her parents to continue competing even though she strongly felt like leaving the sport. When she used cocaine, however, she felt able to master the conflict.

For athletes, the drugs are likely to be used in a social context to make their use more acceptable, as well as to deny the problems motivating the usage. Often, only after considerable examination, are the true factors recognized.

At the same time, alcohol, marijuana, or barbiturates may be used to achieve a tranquilizing effect (although in athletes and college students barbiturate use appears low). The most dangerous coupling occurs when stimulants are used to become aroused or motivated for practice or competition, and then tranquilizing drugs are used to come-down. Again, alcohol or marijuana are likely to be used in social settings, helping to deny the problems motivating the usage.

This combination of *uppers and downers* is both physically and psychologically dangerous and has a strong possibility, with increased usage, of facilitating the development of dependency problems.

Affection and Intimacy Needs

Athletes, often from childhood or adolescence onward, are placed in an environment that encourages aggressiveness, competitiveness, and perhaps less sensitivity to the feelings of others. To an extent, this overemphasizes some of the traditional aspects of the male role in our society, and it is opposite to the traditional female role.

Athletes may not learn how to express their needs to others, or their feelings for others. In some cases, these patterns may be inhibited by an excessive emphasis on the competitive, aggressive, and calloused roles set out for them.

One male athlete, seen in therapy, expressed it dramatically, "The only time I can say 'I love you' to anyone is when I'm stoned."

For some athletes, alcohol or drugs provide a vehicle through which they can express their more tender feelings and needs. Unfortunately, once the effects of the alcohol or drugs wear off, they may not have the ability to continue in this direction.

There is also the problem of *pseudointimacy*. Under the effects of alcohol or drugs, individuals may perceive more to exist than in fact does exist. When the alcohol or drugs wear off, the positive feelings disappear. The only way in which to make them reappear, like spirits at a séance, is through repeated use of alcohol and/or drugs. As can be seen, a deleterious pattern may develop for an individual who has strong needs to experience or express such feelings. Where groups form to express similar needs and feelings, the inability of the individuals to express these needs and feelings in a normal state of consciousness can reinforce the use of alcohol and drugs, particularly when it is subconsciously recognized that without these substances the feelings will not exist.

Implications of the Psychological Factors for Athlete Alcohol and Drug Use

Over two decades ago Nicholi (1967) commented that, while at one time special skills such as athletics may have protected individuals from using drugs by shoring up self-esteem, this was no longer the case. Recreational drugs had found their way into the mainstream, and it was no longer the marginal individual who used drugs. Pope et al. (1981) noted that participation in any college activity, including varsity, intramural, and other sports, in no way related to the use of recreational drugs and alcohol: that is, the rates among students in these groups were comparable to students in general. Gaskins and deShazo (1985), in surveying athletes at the University of Alabama, found 33% agreeing that drug abuse among UA athletes was a problem. Twenty percent of the athletes also agreed that the occasional use of drugs at social events was acceptable (a cross tabulation of these groups was not provided).

This chapter has tried to set forth specific psychological factors likely to relate to athletes' use of alcohol and recreational drugs. As was stated initially, to understand any individual's patterns will require understanding of the individual. This chapter contains key factors, based on clinical observation and reports in the literature, that are most specific to athletes.

Having stated this, the implication of these factors for preventive intervention must be addressed from a similar psychological framework.

Some of the factors cited relate to broad social issues and are difficult to address for society in general, as well as for athletes in particular. What constitutes recreational use is unclear; whether a recreational drug should be legal or illegal is unclear. The mixed messages given particularly to adolescents, about alcohol and drug use, masculinity, and role models, need attention.

Much of the current discussions about athletes and substance use centers on urine testing as a forcible prevention, and on education as a preventive intervention.

Urine testing appears more as a punishment, and behavioral psychology advises that punishment will only suppress, but will not eliminate a behavior. Athletes may control their usage during periods of training or competition, but may resume usage at other times. For those inclined to challenge authority, a variety of alternatives may be sought, such as purchasing clean urine. Even this may not be sufficient. At the time of the writing of this chapter, three amateur boxers had been disqualified at an Olympic trial for urine samples showing marijuana or cocaine, and five professional football players were penalized for recreational drug residue found in their urine.

Murphy estimated that 20% of the athletes at Ohio State University abused either drugs or alcohol, and of these, half would stop only when threatened with suspension or expulsion or, because of their dependence, would not respond to anything (Drug Testing in Sports 1985). Murray, also voices the paradox: why test athletes for *pleasure enhancing* drugs, and not other segments of society? This usage does not have the same ethical impact as does *performance enhancing* drugs.

Murray (1986, p. 48) states, "athletes are often treated like children—large and physically gifted children, but children . . . screening for pleasure drugs is just one more way of telling them that they are not, and can not be responsible individuals."

It must be clear to athletes why they are being targeted for special consideration around the issues of alcohol and recreational drug use. Creating feelings of persecution or minority status is not likely to reduce the factors contributing to usage.

It is important to note that Duda (1984), in reviewing a Big 10 study of male athletes and nonathletes, found 25% of the nonathletes smoked cigarettes—but only three athletes—a minuscule percentage, also smoked. Quite clearly, athletes perceive cigarettes as deleterious to their health and/or performance. It can only be wondered, if reliable and accurate information about other substances were available, would other usage rates drop? It is also likely that the smoking rate among nonathletes is lower than it might have been ten or twenty years ago.

It is difficult to imagine an idolized athlete advertising for money, or personally endorsing cigarettes. This, of course, did happen prior to the 1963 Surgeon General's report on smoking. Would more consistent behaviors around alcohol and drug use by valued athletes slower the usage for younger athletes? Social psychology would lead us to expect so.

Preventive education programs for athletes, dealing only with alcohol and drug use are likely to be minimally effective. Unless similar programs depress use among peer groups, the athletes will still be placed in difficult binds. At the same time, the factors within the athletic environment, including those described in this chapter, must also be addressed. Athletes must be helped to recognize their own needs and conflicts, and to develop more positive paths to self-development and self-esteem. Such programs, not geared simply toward alcohol and drugs, but toward broader issues relating to athletes' personal development, have been described (Heyman 1987; Lanning 1982; Remer et al. 1978; Wittmer et al. 1981). Such programs would far more broadly get at the factors that predispose athletes to substance use and abuse.

This is not meant to imply such programs should be designed for athletes only. If we assume such programs are most likely to be implemented at the high school or college level, it would be ideal for such programs to be developed for students in general. Regrettably, time and money are likely to be limited.

Any program must convey a sense of personal caring about the athletes. It is this writer's view that programs developed to control athletes because of public relations will at best be transient in their effects, and will likely have to rely on punishment for compliance. Programs developed out of sincere caring for athletes as individuals are much more likely to involve athletes personally, and to develop long-lasting insights, and more appropriate behaviors.

Summary

It is hoped that the psychological factors described in this chapter will be of use to individual athletes trying to understand themselves, as well as to those working with, or concerned about, athletes. As so often is the case in writing a chapter, one is left with the unsettling feelings that the complexity of the issues cannot be dealt with in such limited space, and that an entire volume could be devoted to the issues involved. If, however, this is a good beginning place for readers, the purpose will have been achieved.

References

Bandura, A. and Walters, R. H. (1963) Social learning and personality development, NY: Holt, Rinehart, & Winston.

Bell, J. A. and Doege, T. C. (1987) Athletes use and abuse of drugs. *Physician and Sportsmedicine.* 15:99–108.

Clement, D. B. (1983) Drug use survey: Results and conclusions. *Physician and Sportsmedicine.* 11:64–67.

Drug testing in sports: A round table. (1985) *Physician and Sportsmedicine.* 13:69–82.

Duda, M. (1986) Female athletes: Targets for drug abuse. *Physician and Sportsmedicine.* 14:142–146.

Duda, M. (1984) Drug testing challenges college and proathletes. *Physician and Sportsmedicine.* 12:109–116.

Edwards, H. (1987) Sport's tragic drug connection: Where do we go from here? *Journal of Sport and Social Issues.* (10):1–5.

Erikson, E. (1968) *Identity: Youth and crisis.* New York: Norton.

Gaskins, S. E. and deShazo, W. F. (1985) Attitude toward drug abuse screening for an intercollegiate athletic program. *Physician and Sportsmedicine.* 13:93–100.

Heyman, S. R. (1987) Counseling and psychotherapy with athletes: Special considerations. In *Sport Psychology: The psychological health of the athlete,* J. R. May and M. J. Asken, ed. New York: PMA Publishing Corp.

Heyman, S. R. and Rose, K. G. (1981) *The relationships of personality and behavioral characteristics to the SCUBA performance of novices.* Paper presented at the 1981 meeting of the North American Society for Psychology of Sport and Physical Activity, Asilomar, CA., May, 1981.

Heyman, S. R. and Rose, K. G. (1980) Psychological variables affecting SCUBA performance. In *Psychology of motor behavior and sport— 1979,* ed. C. H. Nadeua et al., pp. 180–188. Champaign IL: Human Kinetics Publishers.

Lanning, W. (1982) The privileged few: Special counseling needs of athletes. *Journal of Sport Psychology.* 4:19–23.

Mandell, A. J.; Stewart, K. D.; and Russo, P. V. (1981) The Sunday syndrome: From kinetics to altered consciousness. *Federation Proceedings.* 40:2693–2968.

Murray, T. H. (1986) Drug testing and moral responsibility. *Physician and Sportsmedicine.* 14:47–48.

Nicholi, A. M. (1983) The nontherapeutic use of psychoactive drugs. *New England Journal of Medicine.* 308:925–933.

Nicholi, A. M. (1967) Harvard dropouts: Some psychiatric findings. *American Journal of Psychiatry.* 124:651–658.

Petrie, A. (1967) *Individuality in pain and suffering.* Chicago: University of Chicago Press.

Pope, H. G.; Ionescu-Pioggia, M.; and Cole, J. O. (1981) Drug use and life style among college undergraduates: Nine years later. *American Journal of Psychiatry.* 38:588–591.

Remer, R.; Tongate, F. A.; and Watson, J. (1978) Athletes: Counseling the overprivileged minority. *Personnel and Guidance Journal.* 56:626–629.

Ryan, A. J. (1984) Causes and remedies for drug misuse and abuse by athletes. *Journal of the American Medical Association.* 252:517–519.

Sales, S. M.; Guydosh, R. M.; and Iacona, W. (1974) Relationship between "strength of the nervous system" and the need for stimulation. *Journal of Personality and Social Psychology.* 29:16–22.

Sarason, I. G. and Sarason, B. R. (1984) *Abnormal psychology.* 4th. Englewood Cliffs, NJ: Prentice-Hall.

Smith, G. (1983) Recreational drugs in sport. *Physician and Sportsmedicine.* 11:75–77.

Special report: Drug abuse in sports. (1982) *Physician and Sportsmedicine.* 10:114–123.

Straub, W. F. (1982) Sensation seeking among high and low-risk male athletes. *Journal of Sport Psychology.* 4:246–253.

Toohey, J. V. (1978) Nonmedical drug use among intercollegiate athletes at 5 American universities. *Bulletin on Narcotics.* 30:61–64.

Ugoccioni, S. M. and Ballantyne, R. H. (1980) Comparison of attitudes and sex roles for female athlete participants and nonparticipants. *International Journal of Sport Psychology.* 11:42–47.

Wittmer, J.; Bostic, D.; Phillips, T. D.; and Waters, W. (1981) The personal, academic, and career problems of college student athletes: Some possible answers. *Personnel and Guidance Journal.* 60:52–55.

Zuckerman, M. (1979) *Sensation seeking: Beyond the optimal level of arousal.* Hillsdale, NJ: L. Erlbaum Associates.

CHAPTER 6

DILEMMA OF DRUG USE FOR MAINTENANCE AND REHABILITATION

James A. Hill, M.D.

Introduction

Injury is an unfortunate coincidence of athletic participation. The number of sports injuries is overwhelming. Almost 11 million people each year are injured in the pursuit of fitness and competition according to a special study prepared by the Consumer Product Safety Commission (Southmayd and Hoffman 1981). More than 55 percent of all sports injuries occur in four sports: bicycling, baseball, football, and basketball. Seventy percent of all sports injuries happen to athletes between the ages of 10 and 24. Sixty percent of all sports injuries are either sprains, strains, contusions, abrasions, or lacerations. Football, which is commonly associated with the highest incidence of serious injuries, has an overall likelihood of injury ranging between 11 percent and 81 percent (Robey 1971). Thus, injury is as common to sports as victory and defeat.

Drugs are commonly used to treat athletic injuries in conjunction with rest, rehabilitative exercises, and modalities such as ice, ultrasound, etc. Drugs should only be prescribed by a physician. But, because of the emotional and financial rewards associated with sports, the physician is commonly placed in the difficult situation of treating an athlete who wishes to continue to compete despite an injury. Physicians commonly prescribe drugs when an injury is minor and the medication allows the athlete to continue to compete without risk of worsening the injury or causing a new injury. However, a physician can be considered negligent in prescribing drugs that could cause injury or worsen an existing injury, especially if the athlete has not given his or her consent based upon knowledge of the potential dangers that the drugs might pose.

Commonly used drugs in sports, in the armamentarium of a physician, fall into three major categories. One category is medically called *analgesics.* Analgesic is the medical name for a pain reliever. The second category is *muscle relaxants,* which do what the name implies; and the third category is *anti-inflammatory agents,* which are drugs that decrease tissue swelling and irritation.

Analgesics

Analgesics, or pain relievers, can be divided into two types—narcotic or non-narcotic. Narcotic analgesics are medications which can be addictive. They should be employed only in serious and painful injuries as a temporary emergency measure and under physician control. Nonnarcotic analgesics are the most commonly used pain relievers. They are not addictive, nor do they cause drowsiness, clouding of the mental processes, or a decrease in coordination which the narcotic agents cause.

Narcotic drugs are commonly called opiates because they are derived from poppy plants. Morphine is the prototype of the narcotic drugs. These drugs affect the brain and spinal cord by competing with naturally occurring compounds in the brain to produce pain relief. Narcotics are most effective for relieving moderate to severe acute pain from various causes. They alter the psychological response to pain as well as its perception, partially at a spinal level, and suppress anxiety and apprehension. They act on the brain to produce pain relief without loss of consciousness, but with higher doses they can cause sedation.

The indications for usage are:

1. Severe acute pain
2. Neoplastic disease (cancer)
3. Myocardial infarction
4. Preanesthetic medication
5. Pulmonary edema
6. Cough suppression
7. Gastrointestinal and urinary tract disorders

Narcotic analgesics are used in cancer (neoplastic disease) because of the chronic pain and, especially in its terminal stage, a patient's comfort deserves special consideration despite the drawback of addiction. Myocardial infarctions (heart attacks) are commonly associated with

94

severe pain. Narcotics are used because they provide adequate pain relief without excessive breathing suppression or lowering of blood pressure. Narcotics are useful for preanesthetic medication because their sedative, anti-anxiety, and pain relieving properties afford smoother beginning of anesthesia and maintenance of anesthesia, and they reduce excitement during waking up. Individuals with shortness of breath secondary to heart failure may benefit from narcotics if breathing is controlled. The cough reflex is depressed or abolished by narcotics, but use of strong analgesics for this purpose should be restricted to patients with painful cough that cannot be controlled by non-narcotic drugs. Narcotics can produce nausea, vomiting, and constipation, but they slow the gastrointestinal and urinary tract muscle which can be useful in diarrhea and urinary colic.

Narcotics cause adverse reactions that limit their usefulness: breathing depression, nausea, vomiting, constipation, cardiovascular effects (low blood pressure and slow heart rate), and increased intracranial pressure. Insofar as interactions with other drugs, a narcotic's dose should be reduced in patients receiving other drugs that depress brain and spinal cord function, such as, antipsychotic drugs, barbiturates, and anti-anxiety drugs. Severe adverse reactions have been known to occur to patients receiving both Demerol, a type of narcotic drug, and monoamine oxidase inhibitors which are drugs used in depression. The biggest problem with narcotic drugs is that the patient can become physically dependent (addicted) and develop a high tolerance to the drug. The development of physical dependence and tolerance with prolonged use of narcotics varies from patient to patient. The physician must be constantly alert to certain considerations: (1) the patient may be simulating a disease in order to obtain a dependence-producing drug, (2) the effective dose level will vary depending upon the degree of tolerance; and (3) abrupt discontinuation can precipitate a withdrawal syndrome which is associated with severe illnesses and, in some instances, can lead to death if a patient with an addiction undergoes major medical or surgical trauma. Although it is often difficult to identify dependence-prone patients, physicians should make every effort to do so. Patients who are emotionally unstable, those with a history of addiction or abuse of other drugs, such as cocaine, alcohol, etc., and patients with mental disorders may be predisposed to narcotic abuse. Narcotics use should be monitored very carefully in these patients, but they should not be deprived of necessary analgesics.

Dosage of strong analgesics, such as narcotics, should be individualized and based on the severity of pain. For rapid onset of effect these drugs must be given by intramuscular injection. For a less rapid onset of action these drugs can be given orally. Also, these drugs can be given intravenously to produce a more rapid onset of action with greater dosage control.

Tables 1 through 8, in the Drug Reference Tables beginning on page 102, outline the commonly used narcotic drugs: their indications for usage, contraindications, warnings/precautions, adverse reactions, signs and symptoms of overdosage, drug interactions, altered laboratory values, and other drugs containing the narcotic drug. The mixtures of different analgesic drugs from different classes are among the most widely used drugs. Most of these mixture drugs are formulated on the theoretical basis that they produce a greater analgesic effect, provide broader uses, or cause fewer, or less severe, side effects than a single ingredient.

Non-narcotics

This class of drugs is commonly used to relieve pain, but it also has an effect to decrease temperature and inflammation. In certain instances, these drugs (aspirin, Tylenol, ibuprofen, etc.) can be bought over-the-counter without a physician prescription. How these drugs work is not known. Evidence from animal studies has shown that the analgesic effect of aspirin and Tylenol on pain is principally peripheral, as opposed to narcotic drugs which affect the central nervous system. The primary clinical effects appear to be related to the inhibition of production of hormones in the body called prostaglandins, whose actions include pain, fever, swelling, and redness.

Although the therapeutic actions of this group of drugs may result from blocking prostaglandin production, this property may also produce many of their side effects. These effects include prolonged bleeding times, gastrointestinal irritation and ulceration, and decreased kidney function. Allergic responses, with shortness of breath, rash, itching and swelling, may also occur following a single dose or in patients who have previously received these drugs without any problems.

Non-narcotics are commonly used in mild to moderate pain. Circumstances in which they are commonly used are headaches, muscle sprains, ligament strains, and joint discomfort. These drugs are generally not useful in severe pain. All the drugs in this class are antipyretics, which means they reduce fever. Because of the association of an increased incidence of Reye's syndrome, a potentially fatal disease, with the use of aspirin during the early phase of influenza (flu syndrome) or chicken pox infections, only Tylenol is recommended to decrease fever of unknown cause in children and adolescents. Either drug may be used in adults.

The choice of analgesic drug depends upon the effectiveness and side effects of a particular drug in the individual patient. The most widely used drugs of this class are aspirin and acetaminophen (Tylenol). They are equivalent in analgesic and antipyretic properties, but their actions and side effects differ. For instance, aspirin has a significant anti-inflammatory effect, whereas Tylenol was only a weak peripheral anti-inflammatory activity. Newer drugs, such as ibuprofen (Motrin), Dolobid, Nalfon, Naprosyn, and Suprol, are commonly used as analgesics and anti-inflammatory drugs, and clinical studies show they are as, or are more, effective than aspirin, acetaminophen (Tylenol), or codeine.

Tables 9 through 15 outline the commonly used non-narcotic analgesics: their indications for usage, contraindications, warnings/precautions, adverse reactions, signs and symptoms of overdosage, drug interactions, altered laboratory values, and other drugs containing the non-narcotic pain relievers. Suprol (Table 15), because of the potential for developing flank pain with renal dysfunction, should not be considered as initial treatment for pain and used only after other drugs have failed.

Many products contain two or more non-narcotic analgesics, such as aspirin and acetaminophen. The analgesic effect of such a combination is no greater than the sum of the effects of the individual drugs, and no advantage has ben demonstrated by combining them.

Muscle Relaxants

Muscle spasm is an involuntary contraction of a muscle, or group of muscles, usually accompanied by pain and limited function. Reflex muscle spasm, or splinting, often occurs as a protective response to local injury, but it may be significant and require treatment. Minor injuries and muscle strains usually respond rapidly to rest and rehabilitation. More severe acute or chronic local muscle spasms may be produced by muscle strains and ligament sprains, trauma, and cervical or lumbar radiculopathy (pinched nerve) caused by degenerative osteoarthritis, herniated disc, spondylitis, or irritation from surgery. These muscle spasms are characterized by local pain, tenderness on palpation, increased muscle tone, and limitation of motion. These severe acute or chronic local muscle spasms are the conditions commonly treated with muscle relaxants.

These drugs work by depressing the nerve input affecting muscle stretch reflexes. Most muscle relaxants are chemically related to the tricyclic anti-depressants and produce sedation. Addiction (physical dependence) may develop after long-term usage of large doses of some of the muscle relaxants, especially in patients with a known tendency to abuse drugs. Abrupt discontinuance after prolonged use of large amounts may produce severe withdrawal symptoms, including convulsions.

Tables 16–22 outline the commonly used muscle relaxants: their indications for usage, contraindications, warnings/precautions, adverse reactions, signs and symptoms of overdosage, drug interactions, altered laboratory values, and other drugs containing muscle relaxants. Because they are not effective pain relievers, there are several drugs which combine muscle relaxants with analgesics (e.g., Norgesic, Norgesic Forte, Parafon Forte, Robaxisal, Soma Compound, and Soma Compound with codeine).

Anti-inflammatory Agents

As previously mentioned, muscle strains, ligament sprains, and contusions are the most common types of athletic injuries. In each of these injuries there is an immediate disruption of the primary structures (ligaments, tendons, and muscles) and injury of the associated soft tissue structures (nerves, capillaries, and blood vessels). Depending on the severity of the injury, there will be varying degrees of pain and swelling. The immediate pain is caused by the damage to nerve endings within the primary structures or soft tissues, or both. Immediate swelling is internal bleeding, again due to disruption of the primary or soft tissue structures.

After injury, the body healing process occurs by way of what is called the *inflammatory response*. In the inflammatory response, the blood supply to the injured area is increased to: (1) bring white blood cells to the area of injury to fight off infection and remove dead tissue; (2) bring nutrients into the area to help rebuild the weakened tissue; and (3) bring new blood vessels to the area to increase oxygen, etc. The classic signs of inflammation are pain, heat, redness, swelling, and sometimes loss of function.

The accumulation of blood from the original injury, and the onset of inflammatory fluid, sometimes combine to restrict normal blood flow to damaged tissue cells and may exaggerate the injury. The inflammatory process is mediated by a variety of endogenous hormones, which include the prostaglandins. All effective anti-inflammatory drugs inhibit prostaglandin production. Since prostaglandin production is responsible for the manifestation of pain, anti-inflammatory drugs commonly relieve pain. Steroids are the most potent anti-inflammatory drugs, but because of their significant side effects, nonsteroidal anti-inflammatory drugs (e.g., aspirin, Dolobid, Nalfon, Buprofen, Ketoprofen, Naproxen, Prioxicam, Sulindac, Tolmetin, Meclofenamate, Indomethaciin, and Phenylbutazone) are used primarily for their anti-inflammatory and analgesic activity.

Tables 9 through 15 consist of the non-narcotic pain reliever drugs which are also anti-inflammatory agents. Aspirin is the protype and the most commonly used.

Tables 23 through 29 consist of other drugs used exclusively as anti-inflammatory drugs. These tables outline their indications for usage, contraindications, warnings/precautions, adverse reactions, signs and symptoms of overdosage, drug interactions, altered laboratory values, and other drugs containing the anti-inflammatory agents. As one can see from the tables, these drugs are associated with significant side effects. The three major ones are the effects on the gastrointestinal tract, liver, and kidney. These drugs can cause ulcers, liver failure, and kidney failure, and these systems should be monitored closely. Also, the anti-inflammatory drugs impair platelet aggregation and prolong bleeding time, and should be used cautiously in patients with bleeding disorders. Anti-inflammatory drugs are frequently used by team physicians for early injury treatment to diminish the inflammatory response, which can aggravate and/or increase the injury, and to allow the athlete to begin rehabilitation and return to action sooner. But, it should be kept in mind that the inflammatory response is necessary for normal healing.

Corticosteroids are used occasionally as anti-inflammatory drugs and whether taken orally or injected, are extremely effective. Corticosteroids, however, are in the same class of drugs as anabolic steroids but have very little effect on skeletal muscles. Their effectiveness is different from the other anti-inflammatory drugs: instead of effecting prostaglandin production, they inhibit the inflammatory process at the cellular level.

Corticosteroids are associated with a high number of side effects which limit their usefulness, such as, gastrointestinal disturbances, fluid retention, osteoporosis, osteonecrosis, growth suppression, central nervous system effects—even to the point of physical dependence, muscle breakdown, and abnormal carbohydrate metabolism. Because of these significant complications, oral corticosteroids, with prednisone being the most common one used, are rarely given. On the other hand, it is not uncommon to inject steroids in an inflamed area. This mode of delivery is also very effective and avoids the systemic side effects.

The problem with injecting steroids is that it inhibits collagen crosslinking. Collagen is the basic fibrous tissue which makes up tendons and ligaments. If collagen crosslinking is impaired, healing is also delayed and the structure is weaker for a longer period of time. The problem this presents for the athlete and physician is that the signs of inflammation are diminished due to the injection of the steroid compound, but the healing of the injured tendon or ligament is actually delayed. Because of the delayed healing and weakness of the structure, the tendon or ligament may be predisposed to a more serious injury despite the lack of associated symptoms such as pain, swelling, and limitation of function. Thus, steroid injections should be used with caution in an athletic population because a minor injury can be transformed into a much more severe injury.

Another drug commonly used for its anti-inflammatory effect in athletes in DMSO (dimethyl sulfoxide). This drug is a solvent used in industry. DMSO is rapidly absorbed through the skin and may take other substances through the skin with it. The only approved medical use of DMSO is for bladder inflammation, and it is given by direct bladder instillation. There is no medical evidence that it decreases inflammation, although some athletes swear by it. The most common side effect of DMSO is a garlic-like taste and odor on the breath and skin for as long as 72 hours. This side effect is of no clinical significance. Other possible side effects are skin rashes, allergic reactions, GI disturbances, headache, and vision changes.

Summary

Drugs, in rehabilitation and maintenance after sports injury, are only one component of the overall care of the athlete and should not be looked upon as a panacea. Other treatment modalities, including rest, ice, compression, elevation, immobilization, exercise, etc., are as important and should not be forgotten.

References

Robey, J. M., Blyth, C. S., and Mueller, F. O.: Athletic Injuries: Application of Epidemiologic Methods. JAMA 217:184–189, 1971.

American Medical Association: Drug Evaluations 6th Edition, American Medical Association, Chicago, Illinois, Sept. 1986.

Geffner, E. S. Editor: Compendium of Drug Therapy. McGraw-Hill, New York, 1987.

Southmayd, W., and Hoffman, M.: Sports health, Putnam, New York, New York 1981.

Drug Reference Tables

Table 1   Narcotic

Codeine Phosphate   (Lilly)
Codeine Sulfate   (Lilly)

Vials: 30 mg/ml (20 ml)
Tablets: 15, 30, 60 mg

Indications	*Oral Dosage*	*Parenteral Dosage*
Mild to moderate pain	Adult: 15–60 mg every 4 hrs. as needed	Adult: 15–60 mg IM or SC every 4 hrs. as needed

Contraindications
Hypersensitivity to codeine

Warnings/Precautions
1. Drug dependence
2. Ambulatory patients: Caution patients not to engage in potentially hazardous activities requiring full mental alertness or physical coordination because their ability will be impaired.
3. Patients with head injuries: Usage of drug may depress respiration and increase spinal pressure.
4. Patients with acute abdominal conditions: May obscure diagnosis.
5. Patients with liver and kidney dysfunction: Drug can cumulate in system because it is not detoxified and excreted.

Adverse Reactions (side effects)
Central nervous system: Light-headedness, dizziness, sedation, and euphoria.
Gastrointestinal: Nausea, vomiting, and constipation.
Skin: Itching

Overdosage
Signs and symptoms: Difficulty breathing progressing to stupor or coma, cold and clammy skin, low blood pressure, slow heart rate, and in severe cases, cardiac arrest.
Treatment: Immediate medical care necessary.

Drug Interactions
Other narcotic drugs; sedatives, tranquilizers, alcohol, anti-depressants, and MAO inhibitors: Increase central nervous system depression.

Altered Laboratory Values
Blood/serum values: ↑ Amylase, ↑ Lipase

Other Drugs Containing Codeine

1. Empirin with codeine (Empirin #2 (15 mg), Empirin #3 (30 mg), Empirin #4 (60 mg) Burroughs Welcome
2. Acetaminophen with codeine (Tylenol #2 (15 mg), Tylenol #3 (30 mg.), Tylenol #4 (60 mg) McNeil Pharmaceutical
3. Aspirin with codeine (15 mg, 30 mg, and 60 mg) Generic
4. Phenaphen with codeine (15 mg, 30 mg, and 60 mg) Robins
5. Fiorinal with codeine (#1 (7.5 mg), #2 (15 mg), #3 (30 mg) Sandoz Pharmaceuticals

Table 2   Narcotic

Darvon (propoxyphene hydrochloride)   Lilly
Capsules: 32, 65 MG

Indications	*Oral Dosage*
Mild to moderate pain	Adult: 65 mg every 4 hrs. as needed

Contraindications
Suicidal or addiction prone individuals
Hypersensitivity to propoxyphene

Warnings/Precautions
1. Drug dependence

2. Overdosage:	Excessive doses of propoxyphene, either alone or in combination with other central nervous system depressants, including alcohol which is a major cause of drug related deaths.
3. Ambulatory:	Caution patients not to engage in potentially hazardous activities requiring full mental alertness or physical coordination because their ability will be impaired.

Adverse Reactions (side effects)

Central nervous system:	Dizziness, sedation, light-headedness, headache, weakness, euphoria, minor visual disturbances.
Gastrointestinal:	Nausea, vomiting, constipation, abdominal pain, and liver dysfunction.
Skin:	Rash

Overdosage

Signs and symptoms:	Drowsiness progressing to stupor and coma, respiratory depression, fall in blood pressure, convulsions,, and in severe cases, cardiac arrest.
Treatment:	Immediate medical care necessary.

Other narcotic drugs; sedatives, tranquilizers, alcohol, anti-depressants, and MAO inhibitors:	Increase central nervous system depression.
Anticoagulants: (blood thinners)	Increase effect (increases time to blood clotting).

Altered Laboratory Values
No clinically significant alterations in blood or urinary values.

Other Drugs Containing Darvon

1. Darvocet N50 (Darvon 50 mg plus Tylenol) Lilly
2. Darvocet N100 (Darvon 100 mg plus Tylenol) Lilly
3. Darvon N (Darvon 100 mg) Lilly
4. Darvon Compound (Darvon 32 mg, aspirin, and caffeine) Lilly
5. Darvon Compound 65 (Darvon 65 mg, aspirin, and caffeine) Lilly
6. Wygesic (Darvon 65 mg plus Tylenol) Wyeth

Table 3   Narcotic

Demerol (meperidine hydrochloride)   Winthrop-Breon

Tablets: 50 mg, 100 mg
Vials: 50 mg/ml (30 ml), 100 mg/ml (20 ml)

Indications	*Oral Dosage*	*Parenteral Dosage*
Moderate to severe pain	Adult: 50–150 mg every 3–4 hrs. as needed	Adult: 50–150 mg SC or IM every 3–4 hrs. as needed
Preoperative medication		

Contraindications
Hypersensitivity to Demerol
Monoamine oxidase inhibitors

Warning/Precautions

1. Monomaine oxidase inhibitors
2. Drug dependence

3. Ambulatory patients:	Caution patients not to engage in potentially hazardous activities requiring full mental alertness or physical coordination because their ability will be impaired.
4. Patients with head injuries:	Usage of drug may depress respiration and increase spinal pressure.
5. Patients with acute abdominal conditions:	May obscure diagnosis.
6. Patients with asthma or other respiratory conditions:	May depress respiration.
7. Convulsive disorders:	May aggravate.

Adverse Reactions (side effects)

Central nervous system:	Light-headedness, dizziness, sedation, euphoria, transient hallucinations, disorientation, visual disturbances, headaches, uncoordinated muscle movements.
Gastrointestinal:	Nausea, vomiting, dry mouth, and constipation.
Skin:	Itching and rash.
Genitourinary:	Urinary retention.

Overdosage

Signs and symptoms:	Respiratory depression, drowsiness progressing to stupor and coma, cold and clammy skin, low blood pressure, slow heart rate, and in severe cases, cardiac arrest.
Treatment	Immediate medical care necessary.

Drug Interactions

Other narcotic drugs; sedatives, tranquilizers, alcohol, MAO inhibitors, and anti-depressants:	Increase central nervous system depression.

Altered Laboratory Values
Blood/serum values: ↑ Amylase, ↑ Lipase
No clinically significant alterations in urinary values

Other Drugs Containing Demerol
Demerol APAP (50 mg plus Tylenol) Breon

Table 4   Narcotic

Dilaudid (hydromorphone hydrochloride) Knoll

Tablets: 1, 2, 3, 4 mg
Ampuls: 1, 2, 4, mg/ml (1 ml)
Vials: 2 mg/ml (20 ml)

Indications	*Oral Dosage*	*Parenteral Dosage*
Moderate to severe pain	Adult: 2 mg every 4–6 hrs. as needed	Adult 1–2 mg SC or IM every 4–6 hrs. as needed

Contraindications
Intracranial lesion
Depressed ventilatory function
Hypersensitivity to hydromorphone

Warnings/Precautions
1. Drug dependence
2. Respiratory depression

3. Ambulatory patients:	Caution patients not to engage in potentially hazardous activities requiring full mental alertness or physical coordination because their ability will be impaired.
4. Patients with head injuries:	Usage of drug may depress respiration and increase spinal pressure.
5. Patients with acute abdominal conditions:	May obscure diagnosis.
6. Cough suppression	

Adverse Reactions (side effects)

Central nervous system:	Sedation, drowsiness, mental clouding, lethargy, anxiety, impairment of mental and physical performance, anxiety, fear, dizziness, and mood changes.
Gastrointestinal:	Nausea, vomiting, and constipation.
Cardiovascular:	Low blood pressure, faintness.
Genitourinary:	Urinary retention.
Respiratory:	Depression.

Overdosage

Signs and symptoms:	Difficulty breathing progressing to stupor or coma, cold and clammy skin, low blood pressure, slow heart rate, and in severe cases, cardiac arrest.
Treatment	Immediate medical care necessary.

Drug Interactions

Other narcotic drugs; sedatives, tranquilizers, alcohol, MAO inhibitors, and anti-depressants:	Increase central nervous system depression.

Altered Laboratory Values
No clinically significant alterations in blood/serum or urinary values.

Other Drugs Containing Dilaudid
None

Table 5   Narcotic

Morphine Sulfate

Ampuls: 8, 10, 15 mg (1 ml)
Vials: 5, 8, 10 mg/ml (1 ml), 15 mg/ml (1, 20 ml)

Indications	*Parenteral Dosage*
Severe pain	Adult: 5–20 mg SC or IM every 4 hrs. as needed.

Contraindications
Hypersensitivity to morphine

Warnings/Precautions
1. Drug dependence
2. Hypotensive effect: Lowers blood pressure.
3. Ambulatory patients: Caution patients not to engage in potentially
                                  hazardous activities requiring full mental alertness
                                  or physical coordination because their ability will be
                                  impaired.
4. Patients with head injuries: Usage of drug may depress respiration and increase
                                  spinal pressure.
5. Patients with acute abdominal May obscure diagnosis.
   conditions;
6. Patients with asthma or other May depress respiration.
   respiratory conditions:
7. Convulsive disorders: May aggravate.

Adverse Reactions (side effects)
Central nervous system: Light-headedness, dizziness, sedation, euphoria,
                                  transient hallucinations, disorientation, visual
                                  disturbances, headache, uncoordinated muscle
                                  movements.
Gastrointestinal: Nausea, vomiting, and constipation.
Cardiovascular: Slow heart rate, low blood pressure, and faintness.
Genitourinary: Urinary retention.
Skin: Rash

Overdosage
Signs and symptoms: Respiratory depression, drowsiness progressing to
                                  stupor and coma, cold and clammy skin, low blood
                                  pressure, slow heart rate, and in severe cases,
                                  cardiac arrest.
Treatment: Immediate medical care necessary.

Drug Interactions
Other narcotic drugs; sedatives, Increase central nervous system depression.
   tranquilizers, alcohol, MAO
   inhibitors, and anti-depressants:

Altered Laboratory Values
Blood/serum values: ↑ Amylase, ↑ Lipase, ↓ Lactate
No clinically significant alterations in urinary values.

Other Drugs Containing Morphine
None

Table 6 Narcotic

Percodan (oxycodone hydrochloride, oxycodone terephthalate, and aspirin) Dupont

Tablets: 4.5 mg oxycodone hydrochloride, 0.38 mg oxycodone terephthalate, and 325 mg aspirin

Indications	*Oral Dosage*
Moderate to moderately severe pain	Adult: one tablet every 6 hrs. as needed

Contraindications
Hypersensitivity to oxycodone or aspirin

Warnings/Precautions

1. Drug dependence	
2. Ambulatory patients:	Caution patients not to engage in potentially hazardous activities requiring full mental alertness or physical coordination because their ability will be impaired.
3. Patients with head injuries:	Usage of drug may depress respiration and increase spinal pressure.
4. Patients with acute abdominal conditions:	May obscure diagnosis.
5. Reye's syndrome:	Aspirin may increase the risk of developing Reye's syndrome, a rare but serious disease that can follow chicken pox or influenza (flu) in children and teenagers.

Adverse Reactions (side effects)

Central nervous system:	Light-headedness, dizziness, sedation, and euphoria.
Gastrointestinal:	Nausea, vomiting, and constipation.
Skin:	Itching

Overdosage

Signs and symptoms:	Oxycodone-related effects: respiratory depression, drowsiness progressing to stupor and coma, cold and clammy skin, low blood pressure, slow heart rate, and in severe cases, cardiac arrest. Aspirin related effects: Hyperventilation, nausea, vomiting, ear ringing, headache, sweating, vertigo, flushing, thirst, diarrhea, drowsiness, rapid heart rate, and may progress to confusion, convulsions, coma, and respiratory failure.
Treatment:	Immediate medical care necessary.

Drug Interactions

Other narcotic drugs; sedatives, tranquilizers, alcohol, MAo inhibitors, and anti-depressants:	Increase central nervous system depression.
Anticoagulants:	Increase risk of bleeding.

| Alcohol and steroids: | Increase risk of developing an ulcer. |

Altered Laboratory Values
| Blood/serum values: | ↑ Amylase, ↑ Lipase, ↑ Prothrombin time, ↑ Uric acid (low doses) ↓ Uric acid (high doses) ↓ Thyroxine (T4), ↓ Thyroid stimulating hormone. |
| *Urinary Values* | ↑ Glucose (with clinitest tablets) |

Other Drugs Containing Percodan
1. Percodan – demi (2.25 mg oxycodone hydrochloride, 0.19 mg oxycodone terephthalate, and 325 mg aspirin) Dupont
2. Percocet (5 mg oxycodone hydrochloride and 325 mg Tylenol) Dupont
3. Tylox (4.5 mg oxycodone hydrochloride, 0.38 mg oxycodone terephthalate, and 500 mg Tylenol) McNeil

Table 7   Narcotic

Talwin (pentazocine lactate) Winthrop-Breon

Ampuls: 30 mg/ml (1, 1 1/2, 2 ml)
Vials: 30 mg/ml (10 ml)

Indications	*Parenteral Dosage*
Moderate to severe pain	Adult: 30 mg IV, IM or SC every 3–4 hrs. as needed

Contraindications
Hypersensitivity to pentazocine

Warnings/Precautions
1. Drug dependence	
2. Ambulatory patients:	Caution patients not to engage in potentially hazardous activities requiring full mental alertness or physical coordination because their ability will be impaired.
3. Patients with head injuries:	Usage of drug may depress respiration and increase spinal pressure.
4. Respiration depression:	May result or worsen.
5. Seizures:	May occur in predisposed patients.
6. Acute central nervous system manifestations:	Transient hallucinations, disorientation, and confusion.

Adverse Reactions (side effects)
Gastrointestinal:	Nausea, vomiting, constipation, dry mouth, taste alterations, diarrhea and cramps.
Central nervous system:	Dizziness, light-headedness, euphoria, hallucinations, sedation, headache, confusion, disorientation, weakness, disturbed dreams, insomnia, syncope, depression, tremor, irritability, excitement, and ringing of ears.
Skin:	Itching and ulceration at injection site.

Vision:	Blurred vision, double vision, and nystagmus.
Cardiovascular:	Low blood pressure.
Respiratory:	Respiratory depression.
Hematological:	Decrease white cell count.

Overdosage

Signs and symptoms:	See adverse reactions.
Treatment:	Immediate medical care necessary.

Drug Interactions

Other narcotic drugs; sedatives, tranquilizers, alcohol, MAO inhibitors, and anti-depressants:	Increase central nervous system depression.
Demerol and morphine:	Decrease pain relieving effect.

Altered Laboratory Values

Blood/serum values: ↑ Amylase, ↑ Lipase

No clinically significant alterations in urinary values

Other Drugs Containing Talwin
1. Talacen (tablet, 25 mg pentazocine hydrochloride and Tylenol) Winthrop
2. Talwin Compound (tablet, 12.5 mg pentazocine hydrochloride and aspirin) Winthrop

Table 8   Narcotic

Vicodin (hydrocodone bitartrate and acetaminophen) Knoll

Tablets: 5 mg hydrocodone bitartrate and 500 mg Tylenol

Indications
Moderate to moderately severe pain

Oral Dosage
Adult: 1 tablet every 4–6
hrs. as needed

Contraindications
Hypersensitivity to hydrocodone or acetaminophen

Warnings/Precautions
1. Drug dependence
2. Respiratory depression
3. Cough suppression

4. Gastrointestinal effects:	Nausea and vomiting are more likely to occur in ambulatory patients than in patients lying down.
5. Ambulatory Patients:	Caution patients not to engage in potentially hazardous activities requiring full mental alertness or physical coordination because their ability will be impaired.
6. Patients with head injuries:	Usage of drug may depress respiration and increase spinal pressure.
7. Patients with acute abdominal condition:	May obscure diagnosis.

Adverse Reactions (side effects)

Central nervous system:	Mood changes, sedation, drowsiness, mental clouding, lethargy, anxiety, fear, dizziness.
Gastrointestinal:	Nausea, vomiting, and constipation.
Genitourinary:	Urinary retention.
Respiratory:	Depression

Overdosage

Signs and symptoms:	Hydrocodone-related effects: difficulty breathing progressing to stupor or coma, cold and clammy skin, low blood pressure, slow heart rate, and in severe cases, cardiac arrest.
	Tylenol-related effects: nausea, anorexia, vomiting, abdominal pain, diarrhea, sweating, malaise, and liver disease.
Treatment:	Immediate medical care necessary.

Drug Interactions

Other narcotic drugs; sedatives, tranquilizers, alcohol, MAO inhibitors, and anti-depressants:	Increase central nervous system depression.

Altered Laboratory Values
Blood/serum values: ↑ Amylase, ↑ Lipase, ↓ Glucose
No clinically significant alterations in urinary values

Other Drugs Containing Vicodin
Zydone (5 mg hydrocodone bitartrate and 500 mg Tylenol) Dupont

Table 9   Non-narcotic

Acetaminophen (Tylenol) McNeil

Tablets: 325 mg

Indications	*Oral Dosage*
Arthritic and musculoskeletal pain, headache, menstrual, myalgia, neuralgia, and other painful conditions	Adult: 1 or 2 tablets every 4–6 hrs. as needed
Discomfort and fever associated with viral infections and other diseases	

Warnings/Precautions
Hypersensitivity to acetaminophen

Overdosage

Signs and symptoms:	Early: nausea, vomiting, sweating, and general malaise.
	Late: clinical and laboratory evidence of liver damage (vomiting, right upper quadrant abdominal tenderness, increased SGOT, SGPT, serum bilirubin, and prothrombin time, and possible low serum blood sugar) may not be apparent until 48–72 hrs. after ingestion.
Treatment:	Immediate medical care necessary.

Altered Laboratory Values

Blood/serum values: ↓ Glucose (with glucose oxidase/peroxidase test)

No clinically significant alterations in urinary values

Other Drugs Containing Acetaminophen (Tylenol)
1. Anacin 3 (tablet, 325 mg acetaminophen) Whitehall
2. Panadol (tablet, 500 mg; caplet, 500 mg acetaminophen) Glenbrook

Table 10   Non-narcotic

Anaprox (Naproxen sodium) Syntex

Tablets: 275 mg

Indications	*Oral Dosage*
Mild to moderate pain, menstrual pain, acute tendinitis and bursitis.	Adult: 2 tablets to start, followed by tablet every 6–8 hrs.
Rheumatoid arthritis, osteoarthritis, and ankylosing spondylitis.	Adult: 1 tablet twice a day.
Acute gout	Adult: 3 tablets to start, followed by 1 tablet every 8 hrs. until attack has subsided.

Contraindications

History of allergic reaction to Naproxen

Warnings/Precautions
1. History of allergic reactions
2. Peptic ulcer, perforation, GI bleeding
3. Kidney disease
4. Liver abnormalities
5. Prolonged bleeding time

Adverse Reactions (side effects)

Gastrointestinal:	Constipation, heartburn, abdominal pain and nausea (3–9%), epigastric discomfort, diarrhea, and gastritis (1–3%), bleeding and/or perforation, peptic ulcer with bleeding and vomiting.

Central nervous system:	Headache, dizziness and drowsiness (3–9%), light-headedness and vertigo (1–3%); myalgia, muscle weakness, inability to concentrate, depression, malaise, dream abnormalities, and insomnia.
Skin:	Rash and itching.
Cardiovascular:	Swelling and shortness of breath (3–9%), palpitations (1–3%).
Liver:	Abnormal liver function tests, jaundice.
Kidney:	Kidney disease.
Hematological:	Decrease platelets, red blood cells, and white blood cells.

Overdosage

| Signs and symptoms: | Drowsiness, heartburn, indigestion, nausea, and vomiting. |
| Treatment: | Immediate medical care necessary. |

Drug Interactions

Coumarin anti-coagulants:	Increase prothrombin time.
Lithium:	Increase lithium plasma level
Propranolol, other beta blockers:	Decrease anti-hypertensive effect.
Aspirin:	Increase excretion of Naproxen

Altered Laboratory Values

| Blood/serum values: | ↑ Bun, ↑ Cretinine, ↑ SGOT, ↑ SGPT |
| Urinary values: | ↑ 17-Ketogenic steroids |

Other Drugs Containing Naproxen
Naprosyn (tablet 250, 375, and 500 mg Naproxen) Syntex

Table 11   Non-narcotic

Aspirin

Tablets: 325 mg

Indications	*Oral Dosage*
Pain, including headache, muscular aches, and toothache. Fever and discomfort of cold and flu. Pain and discomfort due to sore throat. Neuralgia, menstrual pain, arthritis, bursitis, tendinitis, and sciatica.	Adult: 1 or 2 tablets every 4 hrs. as needed
Reducing the risk of myocardial infarction (heart attack) in patients with chest pain secondary to heart disease or a prior infarction.	Adult: 1 tablet once a day

| Reducing the risk of recurrent transient ischemic attacks or stroke in men who have had prior attacks secondary to embole. | Adult: 1 tablet 4 times a day, or 2 tablets twice a day |

Contraindications
Gastric ulcer and peptic ulcer symptoms
Asthma
Hypersensitivity to aspirin
Anti-coagulant therapy

Warnings/Precautions

1. Gastric irritation	
2. Patients with blood coagulation abnormalities	
3. Nasal polyps, asthma, hay fever:	May predispose to aspirin hypersensitivity.
4. Reye's syndrome:	There is evidence suggesting that the use of aspirin in children or adolescents with chicken pox or influenza (flu syndrome) may increase the risk of Reye's syndrome.

Adverse Reaction (side effects)

Gastrointestinal:	Nausea, heartburn, epigastric discomfort, anorexia, diarrhea, occult blood loss, hemorrhage.
Central nervous system:	Dizziness, ear ringing, headache, and deafness.
Respiratory:	Hyperventilation.
Cardiovascular:	Increase pulse rate.
Skin:	Rash

Overdosage

| Signs and symptoms: | Hyperventilation, nausea, vomiting, ear ringing, flushing, sweating, thirst, headache, drowsiness, diarrhea, rapid heart rate, convulsions, and in severe cases, may lead to coma and respiratory failure. |
| Treatment: | Immediate medical care necessary. |

Drug Interactions

| Anticoagulants: | Increase risk of bleeding. |
| Alcohol, steroids anti-inflammatory: | Increase risk of GI ulceration drugs. |

Altered Laboratory Values

| Blood/serum values: | ↑ Prothrombin time, ↑ Uric acid (with low doses) ↓ Uric acid (with high doses), ↓ Thyroxine (T4), ↓ Thyroid stimulating hormone |
| Urinary values: | ↑ Glucose (with clinitest tablets) |

Other Drugs Containing Aspirin
1. Alka-seltzer (tablet, 325 mg aspirin with 1.9g sodium bicarbonate and 1g citric acid) Miles
2. Anacin (tablet, 500 mg aspirin and 32 mg caffeine) Whitehall
3. Ascriptin (tablet, 325 mg aspirin, 75 mg magnesium hydroxide, and 75 mg aluminum hydroxide) Rorer
4. Ascriptin A/D (tablet, 325 mg aspirin, 150 magnesium hydroxide, and 150 mg aluminum hydroxide) Rorer
5. Bayer (tablet, 325 mg aspirin) Glenbrook
6. Bufferin (tablet, 325 mg aspirin, 48.6 mg aluminum glycinate, and 97.2 mg magnesium carbonate) Bristol-Myers
7. Ecotrin (tablets, centeric coated, 325 mg aspirin) Smith-Kline
8. Empirin (tablets, 325 mg aspirin) Burroughs Welcome

Table 12   Non-narcotic

Dolobid (diflunisal) Merck, Sharpe & Dohme

Tablets: 250 or 500 mg

Indications	*Oral Dosage*
Mild to moderate pain	Adult: 2 tablets to start, followed by 1 tablet every 12 hrs. as needed
Osteoarthritis	
Rheumatoid arthritis	Adult: 1 tablet twice a day

Contraindications
Hypersensitivity to diflunisal

Warnings/Precautions
1. Peptic ulceration, GI bleeding
2. Kidney disease
3. Liver function abnormalities

Adverse Reactions (side effects)

Gastrointestinal:	Nausea, GI discomfort, and diarrhea (3–9%), vomiting, constipation and flatulence (1–3%), peptic ulcer, gastrointestinal bleeding, loss of appetite, gastrointestinal perforation.
Ears:	Ringing in ears (1–3%).
Liver:	Liver function abnormalities, jaundice, hepatitis.
Skin:	Rash (3–9%).
Genitourinary:	Kidney damage.

Overdosage

Signs and symptoms:	Drowsiness, vomiting, nausea, diarrhea, hyperventilation, increase heart rate, sweating, ringing in ears, disorientation, stupor, coma, and in severe cases, cardiac arrest.
Treatment:	Immediate medical care necessary.

115

Oral anticoagulants:	Increase prothrombin time.
Acetaminophen (Tylenol):	Increase plasma level of acetaminophen.
Indomethacin:	Increase Plasma level of indomethacin.
Sulindac:	Decrease plasma level of active sulindac.
Aspirin:	Decrease plasma level of diflunisal.
Naproxen:	Decrease urinary excretion of Naproxen.
Antacids:	Decrease plasma level of diflunisal.

Altered Laboratory Values

Blood/serum values:	↑ SGOT, ↑ SGPt, ↓ Uric acid
Urinary values:	↑ Uric acid, ↑ Protein

Other Drugs Containing Dolobid
None

Table 13 Non-narcotic

Ibuprofen

Tablets: 200, 300, 400, 600, 800 mg

Indications	*Oral Dosage*
Mild to moderate pain	Adult: 400 mg every 4–6 hrs. as needed
Rheumatoid arthritis and osteoarthritis	Adult: 400 mg 4 times a day
Menstrual pain	Adult: 400 mg every 4 hrs. as needed

Contraindications
Hypersensitivity to ibuprofen

Warnings/Precautions
1. Peptic ulceration, perforation, GI bleeding.
2. Fluid retention and edema
3. Liver function abnormalities

Adverse Reactions (side effects)

Gastrointestinal:	Nausea, epigastric pain and heartburn (3–9%), diarrhea, abdominal distress, nausea and vomiting, indigestion, constipation, abdominal cramps or pain, bloating and flatulence (1–3%), gastric or duodenal ulcer with bleeding and/or perforation, GI hemorrhage, gastritis, and pancreatitis.
Liver:	Hepatitis, jaundice, abnormal liver function tests.
Central nervous system:	Dizziness (3–9%), headache and nervousness (1–3%), depression, insomnia, confusion, emotional lability, drowsiness.
Ears:	Ringing in ears (1–3%), hearing loss.

Skin:	Rash (3–9%), itching (1–3%).
Cardiovascular:	Edema and fluid retention (1–3%).
Hematological:	Decrease white cell count and red blood cell count.
Metabolic:	Decrease appetite (1–3%).
Kidney:	Acute renal failure in patients with pre-existing significant renal impairment.

Overdosage

Signs and symptoms:	Decrease respiratory rate, dizziness nystagmus, cyanosis.
Treatment:	Immediate medical care necessary.

Drug Interactions

Coumarin anti-coagulants:	Increase risk of bleeding.
Aspirin:	Decrease anti-inflammatory activity.

Altered Laboratory Values
Blood/serum values: $\uparrow$ SGOT, $\uparrow$ SGPT
No clinically significant alterations in urinary values

Other Drugs Containing Ibuprofen
1. Advil (tablet, 200 mg ibuprofen; caplets, 200 mg ibuprofen) Whitehall
2. Haltran (tablet, 200 mg ibuprofen) Upjohn
3. Medipren (tablet, 200 mg ibuprofen); caplet, 200 mg ibuprofen) McNeil
4. Midol (tablet, 300, 400, 600, and 800 mg ibuprofen) Upjohn
5. Nuprin (tablet, 200 mg ibuprofen) Bristol-Myers
6. Rufen (tablet, 400, 600, and 800 mg ibuprofen) Boots
7. Trendar (tablet, 200 mg ibuprofen) Whitehall

Table 14   Non-narcotic

Nalfon (fenoprofen calcium) dista

Capsules: 200, 300 mg
Tablets: 600 mg

Indications	*Oral Dosage*
Mild to moderate pain	Adult: 1 tablet every 4–6 hrs. as needed
Rheumatoid arthritis	Adult: 1 or 2 tablets three or four times per day
Osteoarthritis	

Contraindications
Hypersensitivity to fenoprofen
Significant kidney impairment

Warnings/Precautions
1. Peptic ulcer, perforation, GI bleeding
2. Kidney toxicity
3. Liver function abnormalities
4. Prolonged bleeding time

Adverse Reactions (side effects)

Gastrointestinal:	GI distress, constipation, nausea and vomiting (3–9%); abdominal pain, loss of appetite, occult blood loss, diarrhea, peptic ulcer with or without perforation and/or GI hemorrhage.
Central nervous system:	Headache and drowsiness (15%), dizziness and nervousness (3–9%), tremor, confusion, insomnia, fatigue and malaise (1–2%).
Eyes:	Blurred vision.
Ears:	Ringing in ears and decrease hearing (1–2%).
Skin:	Itching 3–9%), rash and increase sweating (1–2%).
Cardiovascular:	Palpitations 93–9%) and tachycardia (1–2%).
Genitourinary:	Bladder inflammation.
Liver:	Jaundice.
Hematological:	Hemorrhage, decrease white cell count, decrease platelet count, and decrease red blood cell count.

Overdosage

Signs and symptoms:	See adverse reactions.
Treatment:	Immediate medical care necessary.

Drug Interactions

Coumarin anticoagulants;	Increase prothrombin time.
Aspirin:	Decrease plasma half life of fenoprofen.
Phenobarbital:	Decrease plasma half life of fenoprofen.

Altered Laboratory Values

Blood/serum values:	↑ Alkaline phosphatase, ↑ SGOT, ↑ Lactic dehydrogenase, ↑ Bun

No clinically significant alterations in urinary values

Other Drugs Containing Nalfon
None

Table 15   Non-narcotic

Suprol (Suprofen) McNeil Pharmaceutical/ortho

Capsules: 200 mg

Indications	*Oral Dosage*
Mild to moderate pain	Adult: 1 tablet every 4–6 hrs. as needed

Contraindications
Hypersensitivity to Suprofen

Warnings/Precautions

1. Gastrointestinal effects:	Suprofen can cause GI bleeding and peptic ulcers.
2. Kidney toxicity	

3. Liver function abnormalities
4. Anemia

Adverse Reactions (side effects)

Gastrointestinal:	Nausea (15%), GI discomfort (13%), diarrhea (10%); GI distress, abdominal pain, constipation, vomiting and flatulence (3–9%); GI bleeding and gastritis (1–3%), peptic ulcers, gastroenteritis.
Central nervous system:	Headache, dizziness, sedation, mood changes, sleep disturbance and pain (3–9%), tingling (1–3%), appetite changes.
Musculoskeletal:	Muscle cramps (3–9%), bursitis (1–35).
Eyes:	Changes in vision and conjunctivitis (1–3%).
Cardiovascular:	Edema (3–9%), hypertension and palpitations (1–3%).
Respiratory:	Upper respiratory tract congestion (3–9%).
Skin:	Dermatitis and itching (3–9%), skin irritation (1–3%), and rash.
Hematological:	Bruising and bleeding (1–3%), white cell count, platelet count, red blood cell count.
Genitourinary:	Urinary frequency (1–3%), acute flank pain with renal dysfunction.

Overdosage

Signs and symptoms:	See adverse reactions.
Treatment:	Immediate medical care necessary.

Drug Interactions

Diuretics:	Risk of renal failure.
Anticoagulants:	Risk of bleeding.
Insulin, Sulfonylureas:	Risk of hypoglycemia.

Altered Laboratory Values

Blood/serum values:	↑ SGOT, ↑ SGPT, ↑ bleeding time
Urinary values:	↑ Uric acid

Other Drugs Containing Suprol
None

Table 16   Muscle Relaxants

Flexoril (cyclobenzaprine hydrochloride) Merck, Sharpe & Dohme

Tablets: 10 mg

Indications	*Oral Dosage*
Muscle spasm associated with acute painful musculo-skeletal conditions	Adult: 1 tablet three times a day as needed

---

Contraindications
Hyperthyroidism
Cardiovascular conditions (see Warnings/Precautions)
MAO inhibitor therapy (see Warnings/Precautions)
Hypersensitivity to cyclobenzaprine

Warnings/Precautions

1. Patients with cardiovascular:	Cyclobenzaprine should not be given during the acute phase after a M.I., or to patients with arrhythmias, heart block, or congestive heart failure.
2. MAO inhibitor therapy:	Do not give this drug with MAO inhibitors, or within 14 days of their use.
3. Mental and/or physical impairment	

Adverse Reactions (side effects)

Central nervous system:	Drowsiness (16–39%), dizziness (3–11%), fatigue, tiredness, headache, nervousness and confusion (1–3%), tremors, disorientation, insomnia, depressed mood, anxiety, agitation, abnormal thinking and dreaming, hallucinations.
Cardiovascular:	Increase heart rate, low blood pressure palpitations.
Gastrointestinal:	Dry mouth (7–27%), nausea, constipation, GI discomfort and unpleasant taste (1–3%), vomiting, loss of appetite, diarrhea, gastritis, thirst, flatulence, abnormal liver function, hepatitis, jaundice.
Skin:	Sweating, rash, and itching.
Genitourinary:	Urinary frequency and/or retention.

Overdosage

Signs and symptoms	Drowsiness, increase heart rate, cardiac arrhythmia, congestive heart failure, convulsions, severe hypotension, stupor, and coma.
Treatment:	Immediate medical care necessary.

Drug Interactions

MAO inhibitors:	Hyperthermic crisis, severe convulsions and possibly death.
Narcotic drugs, sedatives, tranquilizers, alcohol, and anti-depressants:	Increase central nervous system depression.

Altered Laboratory Values
No clinically significant alterations in blood/serum or urinary values.

Other Drugs Containing Flexoril
None

Table 17   Muscle Relaxants

Malate (chlorphenesin carbamate) Upjohn

Tablets: 400 mg

Indications	*Oral Dosage*
Muscle spasm associated with acute painful musculoskeletal conditions.	Adult: 2 tablets three times a day until desired effect, followed by 1 tablet four times a day as needed

Contraindications
Hypersensitivity to chlorphenesin

Warnings/Precautions
1. Mental and/or physical impairment
2. Patients with liver disease

Adverse Reactions (side effects)

Central nervous system:	Drowsiness, dizziness, confusion, paradoxical stimulation (including insomnia, increased nervousness and headache).
Gastrointestinal:	Nausea, epigastric distress.
Hematological:	Decrease white cell count, decrease red cell count, and decrease platelet count.

Overdosage

Signs and symptoms:	Nausea and drowsiness.
Treatment:	Immediate medical care necessary.

Drug Interactions
None known

Altered Laboratory Values
No clinically significant alterations in blood/serum or urinary values occur.

Other Drugs Containing Malate
None

Table 18   Muscle Relaxants

Norflex (orphenadrine citrate) Riker

Tablets: (sustained release) 100 mg
Ampuls: 30 mg/ml (2 ml)

Indications	*Oral Dosage*	*Parenteral Dosage*
Muscle spasm associated with acute painful musculoskeletal conditions	Adult: 100 mg twice a day as needed	Adult: 60 mg IM or IV every 12 hrs. as needed

---

Contraindications
Glaucoma
Duodenal or gastric obstruction
Prostatic gravis
Hypersensitivity to orphenadrine

Warnings/Precautions

Mental and/or physical impairment:	Caution patients not to engage in potentially hazardous activities requiring full mental alertness or physical coordination because their ability may be impaired.

Adverse Reactions (side effects)

Cardiovascular:	Tachycardia and palpitations.
Central nervous system:	Weakness, headache, dizziness, drowsiness, hallucinations, agitation, and tremor.
Eyes:	Blurred vision, increased intraocular pressure.
Gastrointestinal:	Vomiting, nausea, constipation, and gastric irritation.

Overdosage

Signs and symptoms:	Dry mouth, blurred vision, urinary retention, tachycardia, confusion, and in severe cases, deep coma, seizures, shock, respiratory arrest, serious cardiac arrhythmias and death.
Treatment:	Immediate medical care necessary.

Drug Interactions

Narcotic drugs, sedatives, tranquilizers, alcohol, anti-depressants, and MAO inhibitors:	Increase central nervous system depression.
Darvon:	Tremors, mental confusion, and anxiety (rare).

Altered Laboratory Values
No clinically significant alterations in blood/serum or urinary values.

Other Drugs Containing Norflex
1. Norgesic (25 mg orphenadrine citrate, 385 mg aspirin, and 30 mg caffeine) Riker
2. Norgsic Forte (50 mg orphenadrine citrate, 770 aspirin, and 60 mg caffeine) Riker

Table 19   Muscle Relaxants

Paraflex (chlorzoxazone) McNeil Pharmaceutical

Tablets: 250 mg

Indications   *Oral Dosage*
Muscle spasm associated with acute
painful musculoskeletal conditions.   Adult: 2 tablets 3–4 times per day as needed.

Contraindications
Hypersensitivity to chlorzoxazone
Liver disease

Warnings/Precautions
Liver dysfunction

Adverse Reactions (side effects)
Gastrointestinal: GI discomfort and bleeding.
Central nervous system: Drowsiness, dizziness, light-headedness, malaise,
                                        and overstimulation.
Liver damage

Overdosage
Signs and symptoms: Gastrointestinal disturbances, drowsiness, dizziness,
                                        slight-headedness, headache, malaise, or
                                        sluggishness, followed by marked loss of muscle
                                        tone, respiratory depressions and decrease blood
                                        pressure.
Treatment: Immediate medical care necessary.

Drug Interactions
Narcotic drugs, sedatives,   Increase central nervous system depression.
  tranquilizers, alcohol,
  anti-depressants, and MAO
  inhibitors:

Altered Laboratory Values
Urinary   Discoloration (orange, purple, and/or red)
No clinically significant alterations in blood/serum values

Other drugs Containing Paraflex
Parafon Forte (250 MG Chlorzoxazone and 300 MG Acetaminophen) McNeil
  Pharmaceutical

123

Table 20   Muscle Relaxants

Robaxin (methocarbamol) Robins

Tablets: 500, 750 mg
Vials: 100 mg/ml (10 ml)

Indications	*Oral Dosage*	*Parenteral Dosage*
Muscle spasm associated with acute painful musculoskeletal conditions	Adult: 3 tablets 4 timesr per day as needed	Adult: 1–3 a day IM or IV, for up to 3 days

Contraindications
Hypersensitivity to methocarbamol

Warnings/Precautions
1. Epileptic patients
2. Extravasation:Thrombophlebitis and sloughing at injection site have been reported.
3. Concomitant use of CNS depressants.

Adverse Reactions (side effects)

Central nervous system:	Dizziness, light-headedness, drowsiness, headache, vertigo, fainting, mild muscular incoordination and convulsions (injectable form only).
Gastrointestinal:	Nausea, GI upset and metallic taste (injectable form only).
Thrombophlebitis:	(Injectable form only) pain and sloughing at injection site.
Cardiovascular:	Flushing, faintness, low blood pressure, and low heart rate (injectable form only).
Eyes:	Blurred vision, double vision, and nystagmus (injectable form only).

Overdosage

Signs and symptoms:	See adverse reactions.
Treatment:	Immediate medical care necessary.

Drug Interactions

Narcotic drugs, sedatives, tranquilizers, alcohol, anti-depressants, MAO inhibitors:	Increase central nervous system depression.

Altered Laboratory Values
No clinically significant alterations in blood/serum or urinary values.

Other Drugs Containing Robaxin
Robaxisal (400 mg methocarbamaol and 325 mg aspirin) Robins

Table 21　Muscle Relaxants

Soma (carisoprodol) Wallace

Tablets: 350 mg

Indications	Oral Dosage
Muscle spasm associated with acute painful musculoskeletal conditions.	Adult: 1 tablet 4 times per day as needed

Contraindications
Acute intermittent porphyria
Hypersensitivity to carisoprodol

Warnings/Precautions
1. Drug dependence
2. Mental and/or physical impairment
3. Patients with compromised liver and kidney function

Adverse Reactions (side effects)

Central nervous system:	Drowsiness, dizziness, vertigo, tremor, agitation, irritability, headaches, depression, insomnia, and faintness.
Cardiovascular:	Rapid heart rate, postural low blood pressure, facial flushing.
Gastrointestinal:	Nausea, vomiting, hiccups, epigastric distress.

Overdosage

Signs and symptoms:	Stupor, coma, shock, respiratory depression, and (very rarely) death.
Treatment:	Immediate medical care necessary.

Drug Interactions

Narcotic drugs, sedatives, tranquilizers, alcohol, anti-depressants, MAO inhibitors:	Increase central nervous system depression.

Altered Laboratory Values
No clinically significant alterations in blood/serum or urinary values.

Other Drugs Containing Soma
Soma compound (200 mg carisoprodol and 325 mg aspirin) Wallace
Soma compound with Codeine (200 mg carisoprodol, 325 mg aspirin, and 16 mg codeine phosphate) Wallace

Table 22 Muscle Relaxants

Valium (diazepam) Roche

Tablets: 2, 5, 10 mg
Ampuls: 5 mg/ml (2 ml)
Vials: 5 mg/ml (10 ml)

Indications	*Oral Dosage*	*Parenteral Dosage*
Skeletal muscle spasm due to muscle or joint inflammation, trauma, or other local pathology. Anxiety disorders Acute alcohol withdrawal syndrome Convulsive disorders	Adult: 2–10 mg three or four times a day as needed	Adult: 2–10 mg IM or IV every 3–4 hrs. as needed

Contraindications
Hypersensitivity to diazepam
Glaucoma

Warnings/Precautions
1. Mental and/or physical impairment
2. Drug dependence
3. Liver or kidney impairment

Adverse Reactions (side effects)

Central nervous system:	Drowsiness, fatigue, confusion, depression, headache, slurred speech, tremor, anxiety, hallucinations, insomnia, rage sleep disturbance.
Cardiovascular:	Slow heart rate, low blood pressure, cardiac arrest.
Gastrointestinal:	Constipation, nausea, hiccups, salivary changes.
Liver:	Jaundice
Genitourinary:	Incontinence and urinary retention.
Eyes:	Blurred vision, double vision, and nystagmus.
Respiratory:	Coughing and depressed respiration.
Skin:	Rash
hematological:	Decrease white blood cell count.

Overdosage

Signs and symptoms:	Somnolence, confusion, coma, low blood pressure.
Treatment:	Immediate medical care necessary.

Drug Interactions

Cimetidine:	Decrease clearance of diazepam.
Narcotic drugs, sedatives, tranquilizers, alcohol, anti-depressants, and MAO inhibitors:	Increase central nervous system depression.

Altered Laboratory Values
No clinically significant alterations in blood/serum or urinary values.

Other Drugs Containing Valium
Valrelease (capsule, slow release, 15 mg diazepam) Roche

Table 23   Anti-inflammatory

Butazolidin (phenylbutazone) Geigy

Capsules: 100 mg
Tablets: 100 mg

Indications	*Oral Dosage*
Active ankylosing spondylitis	Adult: 1 or 2 tablets three or four times per day
Active rheumatoid arthritis	
Acute attacks of degenerative joint	
disease of the hips and knees.	
Acute gouty arthritis	

Contraindications
Hypersensitivity to phenylbutazone or oxyphenbutazone

Warnings/Precautions

1. Blood disorders	
2. Gastrointestinal effects:	Peptic ulcer, perforation, and severe GI bleeding can occur.
3. Kidney toxicity	
4. Liver function abnormalities	
5. Acute asthma:	Asthmatic attacks may be precipitated in patients with asthma.
6. Rash	
7. Thyroid toxicity:	Hyper and hypothyroidism, thyroid hyperplasia, and goiter have been reported.

Adverse Reactions (side effects)

Gastrointestinal:	Abdominal discomfort and distress (3–9%), nausea, dyspepsia, indigestion, and heartburn (1–3%), vomiting, abdominal distention with flatulence, constipation, diarrhea, esophagitis, gastritis (sometimes with ulceration), ulceration and perforation of the intestinal tract (including acute and reactive peptic ulcer), anemia from occult GI bleeding and hepatitis.
Hematological:	Decrease white cell, red blood cell, and platelet count.
Skin:	Rash (1–3%).

127

Cardiovascular:	Fluid retention (3–9%), edema (1–3%), sodium and chloride retention, congestive heart failure, hypertension, and pericarditis.
Kidney	Blood in urine, renal impairment, and renal failure
Central nervous system:	Headache, drowsiness, agitation, confusion, lethargy, tremors, numbness, and weakness.

Overdosage

| Signs and symptoms: | Mild poisoning, nausea, abdominal pain, drowsiness; severe poisoning, early manifestations: upper abdominal pain, nausea, vomiting, diarrhea, restlessness, dizziness, agitation, hallucinations, psychosis, coma, convulsions (more common in children), hyperventilation, respiratory arrest, hypotension, hypertension, cyanosis; severe poisoning, late manifestations (2–7 days): acute renal failure, edema, hematuria, oliguria, jaundice, ECG abnormalities, cardiac arrest, and anemia. Decrease white count, bleeding disorder. |
| Treatment: | Immediate medical care necessary. |

Drug Interactions

Other anti-inflammatory agents, oral anticoagulants, sulfonylureas, insulin, sulfonamides, phenytoin, valproic acid, divalproex, methotrexate, lithium:	Increase risk of toxicity associated with these drugs.
Barbiturates, promethazine, chlorpheniramine, rifampin, prednisone:	Decrease serum half-life of phenylbutazone.
Methylphenidate:	Increase serum level of phenylbutazone.
Dicumarol:	Decrease serum level of these drugs.
Cholestyramine:	Decrease absorption of phenylbutazone.

Altered Laboratory Values

| Blood/serum values: | ↓ Uric acid, ↑ Glucose, ↑ SGOT, ↑ SGPT, |
| No clinically significant alterations in urinary values. | |

Other Drugs Containing Butazolidin
None

Table 24   Anti-inflammatory

Clinoril (sulindac) Merck, Sharp & Dohme

Tablets: 150, 200 mg

Indications	*Oral Dosage*
Arthritis, tendinitis, bursitis, and other inflammatory conditions.	Adult: 1 tablet twice a day as needed

Contraindications
Hypersensitivity to sulindac

Warnings/Precautions
1. Peptic ulceration, GI bleeding
2. Interference with platelet function
3. Liver function abnormalities
4. Pancreatitis: Sulindac can cause pancreatitis.
5. Kidney   Renal toxicity
6. Aspirin administration: Do not give aspirin concomitantly, as it decreases plasma levels of the active sulfide metabolic of sulindac, has no beneficial effect on the therapeutic response to sulindac, and increases the incidence of GI reactions to treatment.
7. Concomitant oral anticoagulants or hypoglycemia therapy

Adverse Reactions (side effects)
Gastrointestinal: Pain (10%); dyspepsia, nausea with or without vomiting, diarrhea and constipation (3–9%); flatulence, anorexia, and cramps (1–3%); gastritis or gastroenteritis, peptic ulcer, bleeding; perforation (rare).
Skin: Rash (3–9%), itching.
Central nervous system: Dizziness and headache (3–9%); nervousness and ears ringing (1–3%), decreased hearing, blurred vision, insomnia, depression, psychic disturbances (including acute psychosis), convulsions, metallic or bitter taste.
Liver and pancreas:
Hematological: Decrease white cell count, red blood cell count, and platelet count.
Cardiovascular: Congestive heart failure, palpitation, hypertension.
Genitourinary   Hematuria, proteinuria, renal impairment, and renal failure

Overdosage
Signs and symptoms: Stupor, coma, diminished urine output, and hypotension.
Treatment: Immediate medical care necessary.

Drug Interactions

Oral anticoagulants:	Increase prothrombin time
Dimethyl sulfoxide (DMSO):	Decrease plasma level of active sulfide metabolite of sulindac, peripheral neuropathy; avoid concomitant use.
Diflunisal:	Decrease plasma level of active sulfide metabolite of sulindac.
Aspirin:	Decrease plasma of active sulfide metabolite of sulindac, increase incidence of GI reactions.
Probenecid:	Increase plasma levels of sulindac and sulfone metabolite, decrease uricosuric effect.
Other anti-inflammatory agents, alcohol:	Increase risk of ulcer.

Altered Laboratory Values

Blood/serum values:	↑ Alkaline phosphates, ↑ SGOT, ↑ SGPT
Urinary values:	+ Protein

Other Drugs Containing Soma
None

Table 25 Anti-inflammatory

Feldene (piroxicam) Pfizer

Capsules: 10, 20 mg

Indications	*Oral Dosage*
Arthritis, tendinitis, bursitis, and other inflammatory conditions.	Adult: 1 tablet daily as needed

Contraindications
Hypersensitivity to piroxicam

Warnings/Precautions
1. Peptic ulceration, perforation, GI bleeding
2. Interference with platelet function
3. Kidney
4. Anemia: Determine hemoglobin and hematocrit values if signs and symptoms of anemia occur.
5. Liver function abnormalities

130

Adverse Reactions (side effects)

Gastrointestinal:	Epigastric distress and nausea (3–9%); gastritis, anorexia, constipation, abdominal discomfort, flatulence, diarrhea, abdominal pain and indigestion (1–3%); pain (colic), liver function abnormalities,s jaundice, hepatitis, vomiting, gastrointestinal bleeding, perforation, ulceration and dry mouth.
Hematological:	Decreases in hemoglobin and hematocrit (3–9%), anemia, decrease white blood count (1–3%); ecchymosis, bone marrow depression, and nose bleeds.
Central nervous system:	Dizziness, somnolence, vertigo, headache, and malaise (1–3%); depression, insomnia, and nervousness.
Genitourinary:	Renal failure.
Cardiovascular:	Edema (2%); hypertension, exacerbation of congestive heart failure and chest pain.
Dermatological:	Itching and rash (1–3%).

Overdosage

Signs and symptoms:	See adverse reactions.
Treatment:	Immediate medical care necessary.

Drug Interactions

Coumarin anticoagulants and other highly protein-bound drugs:	Monitor patients closely for a change in dosage requirements.
Aspirin:	Decrease plasma levels of piroxicam.
Lithium:	Increase plasma levels of lithium.

Altered Laboratory Values

Blood/serum values:	↑ BUN, ↑ Creatinine, ↑ SGOT, ↑ SGPT
Urinary values:	+ Protein

Other Drugs Containing Soma
None

Table 26   Anti-inflammatory

Indocin (indomethacin) Merck, Sharp & Dohme

Capsules: 25, 50 mg

Indications	*Oral Dosage*
Moderate to severe rheumatoid arthritis, including acute flares.	Adult: 1 tablet twice or three times a day as needed
Moderate to severe ankylosing spondylitis.	
Moderate to severe osteoarthritis, tendinitis, bursitis, and other inflammatory conditions.	Adult: 50 mg three times a day as needed

Hypersensitivity to indomethacin

Warnings/Precautions
1. Gastrointestinal
2. Kidney toxicity
3. Psychiatric disturbances, epilepsy, or parkinsonism: May be aggravated; if CNS reactions are severe, discontinue therapy.
4. Drowsiness: Caution patients that their ability to engage in potentially hazardous activities requiring mental alertness or motor coordination may be impaired.
5. Headache: May occur if headache persists despite a reduction in dosage, discontinue therapy.
6. Infection: Indomethacin may mask the usual signs and symptoms of infection; use with extra care in the presence of a controlled infection.
7. Prolonged bleeding time: May occur due to inhibition of platelet aggregation; use with caution in patients with coagulation defects or in those on anticoagulant therapy.
8. Liver function abnormalities

Adverse Reactions (side effects)

Central nervous system and neuromuscular:	Headache (10%); dizziness (3–9%); somnolence, depression and fatigue (1–3%); anxiety, muscle weakness, involuntary muscle activity, insomnia, muzziness, psychic disturbances (including psychosis), mental confusion, drowsiness, light-headedness, aggravation of epilepsy and parkinsonism, depersonalization, coma, and convulsions.
Ears:	Ear ringing, hearing disturbances, deafness.
Gastrointestinal:	Nausea (with or without vomiting) and dyspepsia (indigestion, heartburn, epigastric pain) (3–9%); diarrhea, abdominal distress or pain, and constipation (1–3%); bloating, flatulence, peptic ulcer, gastroenteritis, rectal bleeding, perforation and hemorrhage of the esophagus, stomach, duodenum or small and large intestine, intestinal ulceration associated with stenosis and obstruction, bleeding without obvious ulceration, perforation of preexisting sigmoid lesions, ulcerative colitis, regional ileitis.
Cardiovascular:	Rapid heart rate, hypertension, hypotension, chest pain, congestive heart failure, arrhythmia, palpitations.
Skin:	Itching and rash.
Liver:	Toxic hepatitis, jaundice.
Hematological:	Decrease white blood count, decrease red blood count, decrease platelets.

Genitourinary	Hematuria, proteinuria, renal impairment, and renal failure

Overdosage

Signs and symptoms:	Nausea, vomiting, intense headache, dizziness, mental confusion, disorientation, lethargy, paresthesias, numbness, convulsions.
Treatment:	Immediate medical care necessary.

Drug Interactions

Diflunisal:	Gastrointestinal hemorrhage (may be fatal); indomethacin should not be used in combination with diflunisal.
Aspirin:	Increase risk of GI reactions; indomethacin should not be used in combination with salicylates.
Probenecid:	Increase pharmacological effects of indomethacin.
Lithium:	Increase risk of lithium toxicity; during combination therapy
Loop and thiazide-type diuretics:	Decrease diuretic and antihypertensive effects; closely monitor therapeutic response during combination therapy. Increase risk of nephrotoxicity.
Potassium-sparing diuretics:	Increase risk of increase potassium and nephrotoxicity. Acute renal failure (with triamterene); indomethacin should not be used in combination with triamterene.
Beta blockers:	Decrease antihypertensive effect; carefully monitor therapeutic response during combination therapy.
Captopril:	Decrease antihypertensive effect.

Altered Laboratory Values

Blood/serum values:	↑ Glucose, ↑ BUN, ↑ Potassium, ↑ SGOT, ↑ SGPT, ↓ Renin activity (PRA).
Urinary values:	↑ Glucose

Other Drugs Containing Indocin
Indocin SR (capsule, sustained release, 75 mg indomethacin) Merck, Sharp & Dohme

Table 27   Anti-inflammatory

Meclomen (Meclofenamate sodium) Parke-Davis

Capsules: meclofenamate sodium equivalent to 50 or 100 mg meclofenamic acid

Indications	*Oral Dosage*
Arthritis, tendinitis, and other inflammatory conditions.	Adult: 1 tablet three to four times per day.

Contraindications
Hypersensitivity to meclofenamate

133

Warnings/Precautions
1. Peptic ulceration, GI bleeding
2. Diarrhea, GI irritation,
   abdominal pain
3. Liver function abnormalities
4. Kidney
5. Decrease white blood cell count

Adverse Reactions (side effects)

Gastrointestinal:	Diarrhea (10–33%); nausea with or without vomiting (11%); other GI disorders (10%); abdominal pain and flatulence (3–9%); constipation and peptic ulcer (1–3%); bleeding and/or perforation, ulcer, colitis, jaundice.
Cardiovascular:	Edema (1–3%).
Skin:	Rash (3–9%) and itching.
Central nervous system:	Headache and dizziness (3–9%), and ear ringing (1–3%).
Hematological:	Decrease white cell count, red blood cell count, and platelet count.

Overdosage

Signs and symptoms:	CNS stimulation, manifest kidney by irrational behavior, marked agitation, and generalized seizures, followed by toxicity, and in some cases, kidney failure.
Treatment:	Immediate medical care necessary.

Drug Interactions

Warfarin:	Increase anticoagulant effect.
Aspirin:	Increase fecal blood loss, decrease plasma meclofenamate level.

Altered Laboratory Values

Blood/serum values:	↑ SGOT, ↑ SGPT, ↑ Alkaline phosphates, ↑ BUN, ↑ Creatinine

No clinically significant alterations in urinary values.

Other Drugs Containing Meclomen
None

Table 28 Anti-inflammatory

Orudis (ketoprofen) Wyeth

Capsules: 50, 75 mg

Indications	Oral Dosage
Arthritis, tendinitis, bursitis, and other inflammatory conditions.	Adult: 1 tablet three to four times a day as needed

Contraindications
Hypersensitivity to ketoprofen

Warnings/Precautions
1. Peptic ulceration, GI bleeding
2. Kidney toxicity
3. Liver function abnormalities
4. Peripheral edema: Peripheral edema has been observed in 2% of patients taking ketoprofen; use with caution in patients with fluid retention, heart failure, or hypertension.
5. Anemia
6. Prolonged bleeding time: Ketoprofen decreases platelet adhesion and aggregation; bleeding time may be prolonged by approximately 3–4 min. from baseline values.

Adverse Reactions (side effects)

Gastrointestinal: Dyspepsia (11.5%); nausea, abdominal pain, diarrhea, constipation, and flatulence (3%); anorexia, vomiting and gastritis (1–3%); appetite increase, dry mouth, eructation, gastritis, rectal hemorrhage, salivation, peptic ulcer, gastrointestinal perforation and intestinal ulceration (rare).

Central nervous system: Headache and CNS inhibition (including somnolence, malaise, and depression) or excitation(including insomnia, nervousness, and dreams) (3%); dizziness (1–3%); amnesia, confusion, impotence, migraine (rare).

Eyes: Ear ringing (1–3%), hearing impairment (rare).
Skin: Rash (1–3%), photosensitivity.
Genitourinary: Impairment of renal function.
Cardiovascular: Hypertension, palpitation, heart rate, congestive heart failure, peripheral vascular disease.
Hematological: Decrease coagulation.
Respiratory: Shortness of breath.

Overdosage
Signs and symptoms: Vomiting and drowsiness.
Treatment: Immediate medical care necessary.

Drug Interactions
Aspirin: Decrease protein binding of ketoprofen, increase plasma clearance of ketoprofen. Concomitant use is not recommended.
Diuretics: Decrease urinary excretion of potassium and chloride. Increase risk of developing renal failure.
Warfarin: Increase bleeding time.

| Probenecid: | Decrease protein binding and plasma clearance of ketoprofen; monitor patient closely. |

Altered Laboratory Values
| Blood/serum values: | ↑ Bleeding time, ↑ BUN, ↓ Sodium, ↑ SGOT, ↑ SGPT |

No clinically significant alterations in urinary values occur.

Other Drugs Containing Orudis
None

Table 29   Anti-inflammatory

Tolectin 200 (tolmetin sodium) McNeil Pharmaceutical

Tablets: tolmetin sodium equivalent to 200 mg tolmetin

| *Indications* | *Oral Dosage* |
| Arthritis, tendinitis, bursitis, and other inflammatory conditions. | Adult: 2 tablets twice a day as needed |

Contraindications
Hypersensitivity to tolmetin

Warnings/Precautions
1. Gastrointestinal effects:	Tolmetin can cause severe GI bleeding and peptic ulcers
2. Kidney toxicity	
3. Liver function abnormalities	
4. Peripheral edema:	Use with caution in patients with compromised cardiac function, hypertension, or other conditions that are likely to produce fluid retention since tolmetin may cause peripheral edema in these patients.
5. Prolonged bleeding time:	Since tolmetin prolongs time, patients who may be adversely affected by this effect should be carefully observed (see Drug Interactions)

Adverse Reactions (side effects)
Gastrointestinal:	Nausea (11%); dyspepsia, abdominal pain, GI distress, flatulence, diarrhea, and vomiting (3–9%); constipation, peptic ulcer, and gastritis (1–3%); GI bleeding, with or without peptic ulcer.
Liver:	Liver function abnormalities.
Central nervous system:	Headache and dizziness (3–9%); drowsiness, depression, ear ringing, visual disturbance (1–3%).
Cardiovascular:	Elevated blood pressure and edema (3–9%); congestive heart failure (in patients with marginal cardiac function).

| Hematological: | Small, transient decreases in hemoglobin and hematocrit (1–3%), decrease white cell count, red blood cell count, and platelet count. |
| Genitourinary: | Urinary tract infection (1–3%), and renal failure. |

Overdosage

| Signs and symptoms: | See Adverse Reactions. |
| Treatment: | Immediate medical care necessary. |

Drug Interactions

| Anticoagulants: | Increase risk of bleeding. |
| Aspirin: | Increase risk of adverse reactions, aspirin should not be used with tolmetin. |

Altered Laboratory Values

| Blood/serum values: | ↑ Sodium, ↑ BUN, ↑ SGOT, ↑ SGPT |
| Urinary values | + Protein |

Other Drugs Containing Tolectin
Tolectin DS (tablet, 400 mg tolmetin) McNeil Pharmaceutical

CHAPTER 7

DRUG ABUSE IN COLLEGE ATHLETICS: THE ROLE OF PREVENTION AND INTERVENTION

Ray Tricker, Ph.D.

Few of the people who are involved in college athletics today would deny that drug abuse presents a serious threat to the ideals of sporting achievement. During the past ten years reports from the media have increased and have expressed a growing concern about drug abuse in sport and athletes who abuse and misuse drugs. According to Burt (1987), drug abuse among athletes has become one of the current potholes in sport which requires immediate attention. Other reports indicate that, depending upon the drug of choice, up to 15% of college athletes experience some personally related problems with drug abuse (Heitzinger 1986). However, this concern about drug abuse in collegiate athletics may not be shared by everyone who is involved. The overall proportion of abusing athletes may not seem to be large enough to warrant great concern, or justify an all-out effort to develop extensive prevention and intervention strategies. However, the magnitude of the problem is serious if we realize that 15% represents a considerable number of talented young people who may be seriously jeopardizing their health, their unique talent, their future in sport, as well as the future of sport itself.

It is important for more and more people involved in sport to know how and why athletes abuse and misuse drugs. A better knowledge of the contributing factors will help us to better understand the magnitude of the problem. However, this aspect of the problem should not necessarily be regarded as the central issue. It is also important to consider two other important questions related to the need for better drug abuse prevention strategies in college athletics. Firstly, what can be done for athletes who have a drug problem? Second, what can be done to raise the awareness of nonusers and athletic personnel to the problem? The second question is particularly significant, since it applies to every person in athletics who can provide support to athletes who have a drug problem and need help. Unfortunately, some may choose to deny that a problem exists, perhaps reassuring themselves that they have no part to play in prevention or intervention when a teammate is having drug related problems. Some individuals do not consider themselves responsible for playing a role in prevention or intervention and prefer to leave any action to others who work as professionals in the field of substance abuse.

The attitude that others can *fix* the problem, can have unexpected and far reaching consequences. For example, a team could be torn apart by a single drug abuser who is resented but tolerated, if a coach chose to ignore the problem and looked the other way. This situation worsens in the light of some reports, indicating that some drug-free athletes have bought drugs for their teammates and have assisted with cheating on drug tests (Burt 1987). These *enablers* worsen an athlete's problem by providing a different, undesirable form of prevention that denies the abuser of important opportunities to deal realistically with their habit. According to Wegsteder "for every person who becomes chemically dependent, there exists a primary enabler, someone who stands between the user and the consequences of the action" (Physician and Sportsmedicine, 1982 p. 118). The far-reaching nature of the consequences of abusing drugs again emphasizes that more efforts are needed by all who are involved in collegiate athletics to address the problem of drug abuse from as many directions as possible.

Fundamentally the development of prevention programs has occurred because it is generally agreed, that prevention of the problem is more desirable than later intervention, which is often costly and involves lengthy attempts to cure drug abuse (Smith 1983; Burt 1987; Bernard 1988). The principal objective of prevention in sport is to encourage all athletes, particularly young athletes, to make responsible, healthy, and informed decision for themselves, based upon the firm resolution that no place exists in sport for misusing and abusing drugs; for whatever reason.

Many positive and determined efforts are currently in progress to prevent drug abuse in athletics. This movement is supported by the belief that good results can be obtained from approaches which include a combination of drug education, random drug testing, a series of well defined sanctions and regulations, and intervention and treatment (Chappell 1987;

Heitzinger 1986). Within the context of the different needs of individual athletes, many initial reports of these techniques indicate that many athletes have been helped to give up or avoid drug abuse. The areas of drug testing, legality and rules and sanctions receive careful attention in other areas of this book. Therefore, the purpose of this chapter is to discuss some additional and important issues related to intervention, and the prevention of drug abuse in college athletics. This involves examining the framework upon which prevention and intervention is based, including some theoretical and practical approaches to drug education and counseling. It is also important to bear in mind that the premise for these approaches is to raise the awareness of as many individuals as possible to the problem of drug abuse in sport, and to encourage more and more athletes to make positive and healthy decisions related to the use of drugs.

Framework for Prevention and Intervention

The concept of prevention and intervention in general, seeks to help individuals to avoid, reduce, and eliminate drug misuse and abuse. This applies equally as well to the abuse of drugs in athletics as it does in any other walk of life. Figure 7.1 illustrates the various types of prevention and intervention strategies which may be considered during the pre-experimental, and more serious chronic stages of drug abuse. Prevention strategies are designed to reduce the supply of drugs, lesson the demand,

Figure 7.1. Stages of Prevention and the Continuum of Substance

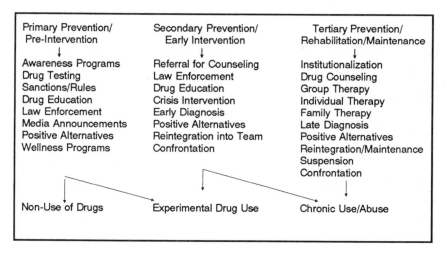

and protect athletes when they choose to use drugs, to avoid the health-threatening consequences of their actions.

Primary, secondary, and tertiary approaches to drug abuse were earlier linked with the community health movement in the 1950's and the 1960's (Kinney and Leaton 1987). For the purposes of athletics, these three different forms of prevention are applicable with efforts which are designed to reduce the incidence of the number of athletes who abuse drugs.

Primary Prevention or Pre-Intervention

This form of prevention is designed to dissuade athletes from abusing drugs altogether, before the experimental stage. This may be less than realistic, because most athletes will have had the opportunity to try drugs at high school and will have already had the experience before arriving at college. However, primary prevention techniques can help these student athletes to clarify their thoughts and opinions about their previous experiences, and give them opportunities to reconsider ways to avoid abusing drugs,

A popular and frequently used method for instructing athletes is through recovering drug abusers as guest speakers. However, a note of caution is needed when considering recovering drug abusers for primary prevention purposes because they could provide a double message to some athletes. The double message may be contained in the perception that athletes form of the recovering person, especially when that individual appears well groomed, healthy and successful, now no longer affected by their previous habit.

The conclusion in the college athlete's mind might be: "Look at him, he abused drugs and he still is a successful, (apparently) healthy person, so why should I worry about my habit? I can recover and do well just like he has." Certainly visiting speakers with a previous history of drug abuse may be helpful in giving the recovering athlete hope for the future, but the value of this form of role modeling for early prevention purposes is questionable.

Other forms of primary prevention may also include: drug education, peer counseling, peer projects, the formation of a strong sense of unity and support within the team framework, and a wide variety of alternatives which have a strong sport psychology basis, including many forms of positive visualization and mental practice skills which are discussed in another part of this book. These prevention approaches should be coordinated with the drug testing program and the sanctions and rules related to drug use which are established within an athletic department.

Secondary Prevention or Early Intervention

Secondary prevention or early intervention measures are necessary following confirmation that an athlete has tested positive for the first time for using an illegal substance. This first occurrence may be treated as an early stage of abuse and often involves referral for diagnosis, counseling, and, where necessary, crisis intervention to prevent further deterioration which occurs with prolonged continuance of the habit. The most important aspect of secondary prevention is to assist an athlete to regain his or her place as an athlete and student, and to establish an ongoing, healthy lifestyle.

Tertiary Prevention, Late Intervention, Rehabilitation and Maintenance

Athletes who have a serious drug problem require specialized, intensive help which involves rehabilitation and maintenance. Such intensive psychophysiologically based treatments usually require athletes to become institutionalized (Moore 1985). The treatment protocols in this setting may include: diagnosis, detoxification from such substances as alcohol and other depressant drugs, individual and group counseling, and group interaction sessions with other athletes who have a drug problem. Following up to 28 days of intensive treatment an athlete would enter the maintenance phase with periodic checks on their progress at a center. Obviously it is important to do everything possible to help an athlete to reestablish some personal goals and a meaning in life. Many athletes have avoided relapsing back into negative habits by providing support as drug educators and abuse prevention counselors for others who are recovering drug abusers.

Athletics and the Public Health Model of Prevention

As an applied conceptual model for understanding drug abuse in athletics, the Public Health Model of Prevention would view the problem as a relationship between the athlete as the *host*, the drugs of choice in athletics (steroids, amphetamines, cocaine, alcohol) as the *agent*, and the sporting arena and the athlete's social background as the *environment* (Wittman and Friedner 1982).

Within the context of this conceptual model, the following factors apply to the athlete (host) in eliminating drug abuse in sport:

- Providing a solid framework of support for athletes which insures the athlete against a *win at all costs* attitude. This requires the support of administrators, alumni, coaches, team trainers, team physicians, and team members. Athletes should not be allowed to compete when any doubt exists regarding injury or sickness.
- Improving interpersonal coping skills; helping athletes to develop a balanced perception of the demands placed upon them as student athletes.
- Encouraging the enablers, who have provided drugs or deny the existence of the problem, to make a positive contribution to an athlete's development.
- Provide more comprehensive educational experiences which make a substantial contribution to the athlete's ability to develop effective decision-making skills.

In relation to the drugs of choice (agent), prevention activities should:

- Demonstrate more clearly that drugs are not *magic bullets*. Apart from the degree of seriousness of the consequences, all drugs produce side effects which may impair or neutralize optimal performance.
- Establish tighter controls over the indiscriminate use of the painkilling drugs (Lidocaine, Procaine, Xylocaine, etc.). By masking pain, these drugs may place athletes at further risk for more severe injury.
- Providing a healthy environment for athletes which involves a social atmosphere that discourages drug use, through improved interpersonal relationships, as well as through rules and regulations.

Within the complex interactions that take place within an athletic organization (environment), prevention activities should include:

- Help for injured athletes so that they still feel part of the team and can continue to contribute to the team's progress.
- Develop clear rules and sanctions regarding the use of drugs during the pre- and post-seasons.

144

- Establish a policy which clearly rejects the excessive use of alcohol consumption as an acceptable way to relax from the demands of sport.
- Encourage opportunities for open and honest communication between athletes and the athletic department as a whole. Develop a strong sense of caring.
- Continue to look for effective ways to deal with stress within the athletic environment.
- Continue to monitor and assist the progress of student athletes outside sport in other areas of their daily lives, e.g., as students.

The effective control of the supply and reduction of drug abuse in sport goes further than the public health model. The abuse of drugs should be viewed as more than just a disease, which can be solved within the context of the host/agent/environment interaction. There is also a great need for effective cooperation, support, and collaboration within the various areas of athletics. As Bernard (1988) has stated: "(Prevention) interventions are collaborative, concerned with providing or facilitating resources to free self-corrective capacities, delivered in a context that avoids the one-down position of many helper-helpee relationships, and sensitive to the culture and traditions of the settings and individuals."

Supply and Demand of Drugs in Sport

Most of the effort to control drug abuse in sport has been directed towards reducing the demand for substances through establishing drug testing programs, drug education programs, counseling, and treatment. Some researchers have also devoted their attention to understanding the sources from which athletes obtain their drugs. Anderson and McKeag (1985) have reported that athletes obtain their supplies of drugs from a variety of sources. The greatest source of illegal drugs came from physicians other than the team physician (25% of steroids), from teammates, friends, relatives, and from public gymnasia. From a historical perspective, attempts to reduce the supply of drugs has presented many difficulties. The drug problems facing society today are sufficient to illustrate the struggles which involve the control of illicit drug trafficking. Answers to the problem of drug abuse in sport will not be found by focusing simply upon closing down sources of supply. More efforts are needed to help athletes themselves decide to reject drug use and start using healthier, more viable alternatives to achieve their goals.

Therefore, more emphasis should be placed upon developing prevention techniques that will deal with the issues from the athlete's perspective. Athletes must be encouraged to become actively aware of the ramifications of substance abuse in athletics. The rewards can be obtained from developing positive coping and decision making skills, and recognizing the importance of clarifying their personal values in relation to drug use e.g., alcohol use. The efforts to educate athletes about self-responsibility and drug use require support from everybody involved in the athletic system of every college. The athlete's support network must place the athlete's health as the top priority; even before the win-loss record. Athletes will care little for drug abuse prevention if a "win-at-all-costs attitude" is the only important factor in their sporting vocabulary. The increasing demand for steroids derives more from a "be bigger and stronger to win" philosophy, than it does from a "joy of competition" approach to sport. Alcohol abuse is another example that can be related to the pressures of sport. The demand in this instance stems from the need to relax or celebrate away from the sporting arena. These and many other issues are important and need to be addressed to fully examine the myths, risks, facts, and fallacies of abusing and misusing drugs. These opportunities can be provided in comprehensive drug education programs, some examples will be discussed later in this chapter.

Theoretically Based Approaches to Prevention and Intervention

The Information Model

Many of the student/athlete-centered programs have evolved from the information model, which has had popularity in the history of attempts to combat drug use by adolescents and children. The inherent assumption is that once informed of the facts, from a personal and legal standpoint, athletes will be deterred from using substances illegally. There is evidence that the presentation of information alone can lead to increases in drug experimentation (Stewart 1974; Pickens 1985). It has also been reported, by evaluators of information based programs, that a greater familiarity with the drug at the informational level reduced negative stereotypes of the drug and actually increased positive attitudes towards its use.

146

The Individual Deficiency Model

This model provides assumptions about an individual's inclination to use drugs in response to some deficiency; an athlete may perceive that through using steroids, that a deficiency in strength or size can be quickly overcome. The programs related to this viewpoint stress improving peer relationships, the ability to communicate with others, and most importantly, developing a positive self-image. This usually involves a values clarification dimension, in which individuals are encouraged to clarify their own values and to reformulate personal values that will be more appropriately self-serving.

The Social Pressures Model

This is a relatively more recent approach to primary prevention. It assumes that an athlete is under a great deal of pressure from peers to get involved in drug use. Anderson and McKeag (1985) reported that friends and relatives were the source of supply from which up to 74% of the athletes surveyed obtained their supply of illicit drugs. In the case of peer pressure, peers may not necessarily be team members but friends with whom an athlete usually socializes away from the team. Therefore, the focus of programs that fall within this model are directed towards helping the athlete to withstand many different forms of social pressure. The term *refusal skills* has become associated with this approach to describe attempts used in counseling and educational programs to teach individuals to refuse invitations from others to become involved using illegal drugs. Encouraging results from this approach have been reported both from the college and high school levels (Severson 1984; Farrell 1987).

The Importance of Family Involvement

The involvement of the family has not been dealt with extensively in relation to prevention. This is important because the family unit may be an essential link to the athlete's problem especially when drug abuse already exists within a family. Another example of family involvement may occur when parents are informed of their son or daughter's drug problem. Heitzinger (1986) has reported that 20% to 30% of athletes surveyed have a family member or parent with a drug problem. For many of these athletes sport provides a valuable outlet, but this may not necessarily help them to completely deal with their inner feelings about the existing problem in their family. According to Heitzinger: "We have to teach college athletes to deal with themselves . . . to take care of themselves, and to not get caught up in the old family roles." Therefore, these athletes will need help learning how to cope with their home situation in the absence of the support group of the team and other friends that they had at school.

When an athlete has a problem with drug abuse, the assumption of a family systems approach is that the athlete's involvement in drug abuse is a reflection of the dysfunctionality of the family. By bringing the athlete together with other family members, a skilled therapist can assist the family in restructuring relationships, opening up blocked paths of communication, and reestablishing positive emotional bonds within the family. A number of treatment programs have reported positive outcomes based upon the effects of family oriented interventions (Levine 1985; Stanton 1979).

Practical Approaches to Intervention and Prevention of Drug Abuse for College Athletics

With the recent increased attention on prevention and intervention, a need for greater diversification and collaboration has been stressed (Bernard 1988). The description of some of the currently reported approaches to prevention and intervention included in this chapter is intended to provide some insight into a variety of techniques that are being used to assist athletes to avoid abusing and misusing drugs.

We might ask: what works and what does not work? This is a natural and common response to the increasing availability of programs at this time. Of course answers to these questions are difficult to find. The reason for this may be found in the fact that most existing programs have not been evaluated to any substantial degree in terms of their impact upon the athletes' behaviors related to drug abuse. The relatively short duration of many programs, and the general lack of evaluative data, provides little insight into what kinds of intervention or prevention methods have achieved success; and equally as important, how success was achieved. In general, impact evaluations of programs in athletics have been derived mainly from self-reports of the organizers and athletes who participated in the programs, rather than from statistically tested results. While most program evaluations do not reveal significant reductions in the uses of drugs by athletes, they do report some encouraging findings in the form of partial successes.

For example, the partial success of a drug education program can be observed in different ways: helping an athlete to realize that he or she has a drug problem; increasing the overall awareness of athletes to the problem of drug abuse in sport; helping to affect the attitude of enablers, so that they refuse to help by supporting an athlete's drug habit by supplying drugs or covering up for the athlete. Behaviors are notoriously difficult to change, and programs often do not succeed in producing immediate changes in behavior. However, this should not stop those involved in organizing prevention programs from continuing to be encouraged by the positive trends mentioned above.

Drug Education

A comprehensive drug education program should form an important part of any developmental approach to prevention (National Institute on Alcohol Abuse and Alcoholism 1984). Athletes need opportunities to evaluate and develop their own perceptions about drug abuse in sport. Ideally, they need to examine the consequences of their actions, and wherever possible without having to experience them directly. Unfortunately, a comprehensive approach to education for athletes has received minor attention in many institutions. Ryan (1984) stated in relation to drug education that: "education of athletes against drug misuse and abuse may have been inadequate and ineffective. But we must continue it and do it better." Ryan's comments were substantiated in a study of forty-four NCAA schools, which reported that drug education received infrequent attention in 95% of these institutions. Only five percent offered any form of regular educational meetings, most of which were predominantly informational (Tricker and Cook 1989). Other research findings have indicated that information alone, and using scare tactics, has done little to relieve society of the problem. In fact in some cases, it actually increased the incidence of experimental drug use (Schaps et al. 1981). The information approach alone has had little success within society as a whole, so is it reasonable to expect athletes to react any differently? With this in mind, Gonzalez (1982) and Goodstadt (1986) have emphasized that, to be effective, comprehensive drug education should be based upon a "knowledge-attitude-behavior change" model which will allow individuals to carefully examine the issues from their own perspective and consider those decisions which best suit their own lives.

149

Effective Drug Education

Effective comprehensive drug education is essentially a function of: (a) the quality of instruction, and (b) the length and frequency with which athletes can be involved with the information, activities, and (c) the strategies designed to encourage effective decision-making, positive attitudes, and healthy behavioral choices. Schaps et al. (1981) reported that 57% of 127 drug education programs, in a variety of education settings, were ineffective because they were too short. Based upon these findings, a *one shot* presentation given by a visiting speaker has little chance of having a substantially positive effect upon athletes. Although athletes and athletic departments follow very busy agenda, it must still be realized that more time and effort must be allocated to the task of educating athletes about drug abuse to produce any worthwhile results. Insights need positive reinforcement, and time should be given to allow discussion and further analysis of the issues. Understanding why an athlete abuses drugs requires more attention than infrequent, single presentations allow. From a theoretical standpoint, one shot presentations given by strangers probably prepare athletes to deal with drug abuse issues as thoroughly as one training session per year would prepare them adequately for the national championships.

Affective Drug Education

Affective drug education strives to foster emotional development, strengthening self-esteem and improving individual and interpersonal communication skills (National Institute on Alcohol Abuse and Alcoholism 1981). Athletes need opportunities to express their feelings in an unthreatening atmosphere, and to improve their ability to communicate with each other about drug use. Athletic departments can contribute significantly to this process by striving to provide an environment which contributes to the total well-being of athletes. Affective drug education is an important supplementary support factor to the athletic environment and can assist both athletes who have a drug problem as well as those who are non-users. In summary, aspects of an effective drug education program can include:

- *Values clarification*—Assessing the alternative to drugs and making informed choices based upon clearly established values.
- *Self-esteem development*—Learning to accept feelings of joy, anger, fear, disappointment; sharing aspects of the self with other

team members; encouraging respect and acceptance of the differences.

- *Role playing*—Through simulated experiences, learning to understand problem situations or value conflicts. Athletes can be provided with opportunities to emphasize with others in a variety of different situations as peer advisors and counselors.
- *Decision making*—Following a close examination of drug abuse issues, problems, solutions, and a sharing of feelings and communication, athletes can be encouraged to make responsible decisions and to express them to their peers in group support sessions.
- *Problem solving*—Involves defining a problem or conflict and listing possible choices or alternative ways of solving the problem situation; investigating the consequences of the decision and establishing the most acceptable outcome for the athlete and team as a whole.
- *Peer advising*—Provides peer advisors for helping other athletes, while having the opportunity to examine their own feelings; advisors can grow and contribute to their own growth, as well as to the growth of others.
- *Role modeling*—As role models, athletes can prepare to make presentations about drug abuse to schools, communities and to peers; opportunities exist for internalizing and examining the issues and gaining a clearer understanding of the problems associated with substance abuse.

Obviously the above strategies have to be carefully incorporated into the busy schedules of athletes to make a worthwhile contribution. Therefore, it is important to consider how drug education can be integrated into a drug abuse prevention program.

Integrating Drug Education into a Drug Abuse Prevention Program for Athletes

A well designed, well implemented drug education program can make an important contribution in helping athletes make responsible and healthy decisions in relation to drug misuse and abuse. At the same time, it must be realized that it can only make a contribution when it is effectively combined with other prevention methods. Voy (Cowart 1988) stated, "drug education, in and of itself will not work. Without testing nobody's going to listen to education." In contrast to Voy, Heitzinger, athletic director and coach (1985) considered, "drug testing is not enough. All it does is to identify the problem . . . it does not solve it." Based upon the insignificant amount of time many colleges have devoted to education, Voy's comments have some validity at the present time. There is much room for improvement in educational approaches. Time alone will reveal if the same comments will also apply to a comprehensive approach to drug education. For the present, the existing negative conclusions about drug education simply reemphasize that insufficient attention has been given to educating athletes about drug abuse in sport. In providing more effective drug education, the following factors should be considered:

- Encourage coaches, athletic administrators, trainers, team physicians, and health educators to participate in the educational process and join athletes in the examination of drug use in sport.
- Consistently and accurately evaluate the combined and separate effects of drug testing, rules and regulations, and drug education upon the drug use behaviors of athletes.
- Collaborate with other institutions to examine more effective ways to educate athletes, and to consider the prevention process.
- Create opportunities for athletes to share their positive perceptions developed from drug education, where they can be perceived as positive role models e.g., in schools and in the community.

Apart from the other forms of prevention which are currently used to deter athletes from abusing drugs, education has the opportunity to touch the ideals of athletes in a positive way, reinforce a belief in the unique worth of every individual, and allow time for sharing of feelings and communication on many levels. Unfortunately in the cases of some athletes, the overwhelming desire to succeed has been negatively reinforced by some people. Whenever fundamental aspects, like reinforcing ideals and communication, have been successfully accomplished by those enablers, they succeed in educating athletes to use drugs, placing the athlete's health and career in sport at risk. We might ask: if education can be successful in a negative way, why will it not work from a positive standpoint? Perhaps the answer to this question lies in the degree to which every participant in sport, athletes and others, is prepared to exceed, in every way, the zeal of drug users and drug suppliers.

Student Centered Programs

Since 1981 Heitzinger and Associates have worked with athletes to provide drug education; assist athletic administrators with policies and procedures related to drug abuse; assist friends and relatives of athletes with drug problems; encourage athletes to confront abuse situations on teams; and assist athletes coming from drug abusing families (Heitzinger 1986). The results of their survey, conducted from 1981–1986 with 9,891 college athletes, indicated that 80% of the athletes do not abuse drugs. Of the remaining 20%, comprehensive drug education and effective policies deter about 5% of users from experimenting with drugs; drug testing and a knowledge of the punitive outcomes deter 5% of the social users, and 5% of the abusers are deterred by drug testing and punishment with counseling. The remaining 5%, the addicted athletes, cannot stop abusing drugs by themselves and need residential treatment, rehabilitation, and maintenance programs with periodic checks.

Combined Drug Education, Drug Testing and Counseling

A 1987 report of the DETER program used at Temple University indicated that $150,000 was invested annually in a drug prevention program for athletes. The program included drug testing, but focused principally upon counseling. The athlete-counselor relationship formed the central focus of the program, with each athlete meeting the counselor twice each semester, once in a large group and once in a smaller group. When necessary, individual counseling provided an atmosphere of strict confidentiality where an athlete could share personal problems and concerns (Farrell 1987).

Since 1985 three athletes have tested positive for steroid use, and during the random testing conducted in 1987 on 350 athletes, no drug use was detected. These results were used as indicators of the success of the program.

NCAA Drug Education Projects

At the national level, the NCAA reported that $430,000 was to be spent on drug education for college athletes as a supplementary prevention project in addition to the existing drug testing policy (Chronicle of Higher Education 1987). The structure of the drug education program included establishing a panel of speakers, whose task would be to provide presentations on drug abuse in sport for universities throughout the U.S.; media coverage and broadcasts on TV in the form of commercial and public announcements during national sporting events, and the development of a series of educational videotapes for distribution to NCAA affiliated university athletic departments on the abuse of alcohol and other drugs.

Wake Forest Drug Education and Counseling Project

The Wake Forest drug education, drug testing, and counseling project involved the athletic department and university officials in a collaborative effort to develop a strong drug abuse prevention program. The program included three objectives: (1) to educate athletes about drug abuse, (2) to deter drug abuse, and (3) to maintain the integrity of the athletic program by identifying and, if necessary, eliminating the presence of the chronic drug abuser from the team (Rovere; Haupt; and Yates 1986). The program did not include any punitive objectives.

The evaluation of the project involved an open discussion session between the substance abuse coordinator and athletic representatives of each sport at the university. The representatives reported that the program had successfully eliminated most recreational drug use and had successfully enabled athletes to resist peer pressure to use drugs at various social activities.

Peer Counseling Programs

Bernard (1988) has referred to peer counseling programs for the adolescent and post-adolescent age groups as the "Lodestone to Prevention." She considers that peer oriented programs facilitate the prevention of drug abuse by empowering individuals with a real sense of participation in solving problems. At the same time, they can develop an increased sense of control and a feeling of responsibility. The extent to which peer programs can positively impact athletes is not fully understood, since the programs, in general, have not produced evaluative data to any degree. However, reports of the success of adolescent and high school based programs are encouraging (Severson 1984; Oster 1983). No evaluative data is currently available to indicate the extent to which this form of prevention can be effective with athletes.

Treatment and Rehabilitation

There are no simple solutions to the many complex problems related to chemical dependency and drug abuse. The extent of recent accounts given by recovering athletes clearly indicates the uphill struggle that faces every victim of drug abuse who goes through a treatment and recovery program. There are many residential facilities around the country which provide care for individuals with dependency problems. An athlete with a drug dependency problem is no different from any other person with a drug problem, and therefore follows similar treatment protocols. As one of the largest publishers in the U.S. of information on chemical dependency, the Hazelden Foundation provides extensive facilities for residential treatment and rehabilitation (Moore 1983). The philosophy for treating athletes with drug problems does not differ from that for any other individual.

The program is geared towards disregarding the athletic image of the individual, to alleviate the *celebrity* status, so that the issue of chemical dependency can be more clearly examined. Athletes are treated as individuals and not as separate types of individuals. During the average stay (twenty-eight days) in the preliminary rehabilitation program, the athlete would follow a tightly structured daily program of lectures and group sessions. By experiencing different situations, athletes are drawn into unfamiliar relationships and become confronted with different problems. With the help that they receive from a support group, many are able to accept and deal with their problem.

Decision-Making and Role Modeling Prevention Program

The DROPP program at the University of Kansas was established, with collaboration of the athletic department and other personnel at the university, to educate athletes about the truths, myths, and risks related to drug use and misuse. The focus of the program was to provide athletes with opportunities for expressing feelings about drug use, developing skills to communicate their feelings, and to experience the part athletes can play as positive role models for others.

The basic premise of the program rests on helping athletes to make wise and healthy decisions about drugs. Most athletes, according to current information, will have had many opportunities to experiment with drugs during their high school years, therefore pure primary prevention is considered inappropriate at the college level. The objective is to raise the awareness of athletes and to encourage a greater sense of responsibility towards the self and their team members.

Evaluation of the program was based upon self-report data collected from the athletes. The results indicated that 95% of the athletes were positively affected. They felt that their experiences contributed significantly to their understanding of many of the problems of drug abuse, and had helped them to make healthier decisions regarding the use of drugs.

The Role of the Coach and Athlete in Preventing Drug Abuse

The success of any program depends upon cooperation and support from coaches and athletes. Without this support even the most extensive and progressive prevention and intervention programs cannot succeed. Athletes and coaches need to be willing to spend time to be aware of precursors to the drug abuse problem. More specifically, they may be able to avoid later, and more serious, situations by being aware and offering help to a team member experiencing difficulties trying to maintain the high standards expected of a student-athlete. The symptoms of drug use vary widely, but if disregarded may lead to more serious, chronic problems. The U.S. Olympic Committee on Substance Abuse, Research and Education (1987) has published the following guidelines for recognizing the symptoms of drug abuse:

- Unusually secretive behavior, especially on the telephone.
- Extreme mood swings from sullen to oversensitive, easily provoked, aggressive behavior, irritable, unaffectionate, uncooperative, and hostile.
- Loss of interest in school, sports, or practice.
- Increased lateness and/or absence from work, school, or practice.
- New and peculiarly different circle of friends.
- Noticeable loss of weight.
- Always out of money. Need for increasing amounts of money. Shoplifting accusations, stealing, etc.
- Avoiding responsibilities, chores, frequently returning home late when expected earlier, missing meals and important occasions.
- Deterioration and change in dress, physical appearance, and interests.
- Refusing to discuss friends and strongly denying or defending issues relating to drug use and abuse.

- Beginning to show mental deterioration, disordered thinking, heightened sensitivity to taste, touch, or smell.
- Paranoid behavior. Insists parents and/or teachers are unfair. Claims others are telling.

Athletes and coaches spend a great amount of time together, and therefore are in an important position to notice unusual changes in a team member and offer help when possible. Although they would like to offer help, many athletes feel uncomfortable about approaching a team member about possible drug use. However difficult it may appear, some situations can be considerably improved when someone cares and offers some help. Thompson, Young, and Grassard (1986) offered the following suggestions in this regard.

1. *Have the Courage to Say Something*
   Try to overcome personal fears and feelings and remain objective, even though the team member may be defensive or angry.

2. *Confront with Facts—Not Feelings*
   Avoid angry confrontations and confront an individual with the facts as they have been observed.

3. *Be Sure to Communicate a Caring Attitude*
   Show genuine concern. Idle curiosity will simply create greater distance from the issues and ruin any positive interaction which can take place.

4. *Know Where to Go for Help*
   Take the time to know where further help can be found. Become familiar with the available resources on campus; counseling assistance, and physicians specializing in drug abuse problems.

Summary

If we can place any value upon current media attention to drug abuse in sport, it is clear that more well organized effort is needed to deal with the problem of drug abuse among student athletes. Awareness of the problem has grown rapidly since the first testing of amateur athletes at the Pan American Games in Caracas, Venezuela, in 1983. Although increasing amounts of time and effort are being directed toward finding solutions, the dilemma which faces sport as a result of drug abuse and misuse shows no sign of diminishing. As we face the future, perhaps the leadership for dealing with this problem will not come so much from coaches and athletes, as from a comparatively small group of individuals who are less directly involved in the firing line of athletic competition. Nevertheless, the ultimate outcome of any efforts to prevent drug abuse in college athletics, will be closely related to the degree to which coaches and athletes are aware of the problems related to substance abuse and are willing to participate in efforts to solve them. There is a limit to which the problem can be discussed here. However, the essential practical elements of prevention and intervention have been well articulated by writers in the field (Crowley 1984; Heitzinger 1986; Burt 1987; Bernard 1988). These aspects are embodied in the comments of Bernard, who has clearly indicated that the essential components of successful prevention involve: becoming individually more aware of the precursing factors which influence drug use; improving the network of collaboration between governing bodies, administrators, and in this case coaches and athletes, and striving continuously to maintain open channels of communication between different organizational groups.

These recommendations provide a feasible solution to the problem of drug abuse in sport. But simply knowing how to prevent substance abuse in athletics is not enough. Active support for long-term prevention efforts is needed from the collaborative efforts of every person who is involved in collegiate athletics.

The importance of developing long-term efforts to solve the problem of drug abuse by student athletes cannot be overemphasized. This is poignantly outlined when we consider the general tendency of people and organizations to respond to crisis with short-term measures. This aspect of human nature has long been a barrier to prevention programming (Bernard 1988). For this reason, current prevention efforts should be regarded as small—but important—beginnings towards the significant contribution that is needed to preserve the special and unique opportunities that sporting involvement can offer. Hopefully, we will continue to acknowledge that the ideals embodied in untarnished sporting excellence have been handed down to us by many outstanding athletes, and are surely worth preserving.

References

Anderson, W. A., and McKeag, D. B. (1985) *The substance use and abuse habits of college athletes.* Michigan State University College of Human Medicine. NCAA Athletic Association Council Executive Committee. Drug Education Committee.

Athletic Director and Coach (1985) *A new perspective on athletes' drug problems.* 3(9):1–2.

Bernard, B. (1988) Peer programs: The lodestone to prevention. *Prevention Forum* Jan:6–12.

Burt, J. J. (1987) Drugs and the modern athlete: The legacy of Lennie Bias and Don Rogers. *Journal of Physical Education Recreation and Dance,* May/June: 74–79.

Chappell, J. N. (1987) Drug use and abuse in athletics. In *Sport Psychology: The Psychological Health of the Athlete,* ed. J. R. May, and M. J. Asken. New York: PMA Publishing Corp.

Chronicle of Higher Education (1987) Drug education to play a major role in ending drug abuse, NCAA believes. Feb.:35–36.

Cowart, V. S. (1988) Drug testing programs face legal snags and challenges. *Physician and Sportsmedicine.* 16(2):165–173.

Crowley, J. F. (1984) *Alliance for change: A plan for community action on adolescent drug abuse.* Community Intervention, Inc. Minneapolis, MN 55415.

Farrell, C. S. (1987) Temple's model drug education program includes tests but emphasizes counseling. *Chronicle of Higher Education* Feb.: 35–36.

Gonzalez, G. M. (1982) Alcohol education can prevent alcohol problems: A summary of some unique research findings. *Journal of Alcohol and Drug Education* 27(30):2–11.

Goodstadt, M. S. (1986) School-based drug education in North America: What is Wrong? What can be done? *Journal of School Health* 56(7):278–281.

Heitzinger, R., and Associates (1986) Data collection and analysis: High school, college, and professional athletes alcohol and drug survey. Heitzinger and Associates, 333 W. Miflin, Madison, WI 53703.

Kinney., J. and Leaton, G. (1987) *Loosening the grip: A handbook of alcohol information.* St. Louis: Times Mirror/Mosby College Publishing.

Levine, B. 91985) Adolescent substance abuse: Toward an integration of family systems and individual adaptation theories. *American Journal of Family Therapy* 13(2):3–.16.

Moore, M. (1983) Hazelden: Putting athletes' drug abuse in perspective. *Physician and Sportsmedicine* 11(12):36–40.

National Institute on Alcohol Abuse and Alcoholism (1984) *Prevention plus: Involving schools, parents, and the community in alcohol and drug education.* U.S. Department of Health and Human Services. Public Health Service. (Washington: *U.S. Government Printing Office*).

Oster, R. A. (1983) Peer counseling: Drug and alcohol abuse prevention. *Journal of Primary Prevention* 3(3): 188–199.

Pickins, K. (1985) Drug education: The effects of giving information. *Journal of Alcohol and Drug Education* 30:32–44.

Rovere, G. D.; Haupt, H. A.; and Yates, C. S. (1986) Drug testing in a university athletic program: Protocol and implementation. *Physician and Sportsmedicine* 14(4):69–76.

Ryan, A. J. (1984) Drugs and self-confidence. *Physician and Sportsmedicine* 11(11):42.

Schaps, E.; Di Bartolo, R.; Moskowitz, J.; Pulley, C.; and Churgins, S. (1981) A review of 127 drug abuse prevention program evaluations. *Journal of Drug Issues* Winter: 17–43.

Severson, H. H. (1984) Adolescent social drug use: School prevention program. *School Psychology Review* 13(2);150–161.

Smith, G. (1983) Recreational drugs in sports. *Physician and Sportsmedicine* 1(9):75–82.

Stanton, M. (1979) Family treatment approaches to drug abuse problems: A review. *Family Process* 18:251–280.

Stewart (1974) Teaching facts about drugs: Pushing or preventing? *Journal of Educational Psychology* 66:189–201.

Thompson, C.; Young, B.; and Gressard, C. (1986) *Cocaine and the student athlete.* Creative Media. 123 Fourth Street, N.W., Charlottesville, VA 22901.

Tricker, R., and Cook, D. (Winter, 1989) The current status of drug intervention and prevention in college athletic programs *Journal of Alcohol and Drug Education* 34(2); 38–45.

United States Olympic Committee (1987) *USOC drug control program.* Committee on Substance Abuse Research and Education, 1–13.

Wegsteder, S. (1982). Drug abuse in sports: Denial fuels the problem. A special report. *Physician and Sportsmedicine* 10(4), 118.

Wittman, F. D. and Friedner, D. (1982). *Current Status of Research Demonstration Programs in the Primary Prevention of Alcohol Problems. Prevention, Intervention and Treatment. Concerns and Models* pp. 5–6. Alcohol and Health Monograph No. 3, NIAAA. Washington: U.S. Government Printing Office.

CHAPTER 8

DRUG TESTING: HISTORY, PHILOSOPHY, AND RATIONALE

James Merdink, Pharm.D. and Bruce Woolley, Ph.D.

Introduction

The misuse of performance enhancing drugs in athletics has been a problem throughout the history of sports. Athletes used drugs and potions to enhance performance since the early days of the Olympics. Ancient literature mentions the banning of certain potions as unfair competition by the early Greeks. During the last few decades, technological advancements in analytical chemistry have made it possible to test for and monitor drug abuse.

The rise of the pharmaceutical industry in the 1950's led to the availability of many new drugs. The most abused drugs in this decade were of the stimulant class; amphetamines and related compounds. Rumors of drug use among athletes and the death of a cyclist in the 1960 Olympics prompted worldwide concern about substance abuse. In 1965, at the first International Doping Symposium held in Uriage, Belgium, Regulation 27 was adopted providing for procedures to curb the drug abuse problem (Percy 1978). The first testing was performed in England in 1965 at the Tour of Britain. This was the first event at which modern, sensitive equipment and procedures were employed. The result was the disqualification of three athletes for amphetamine abuse (Beckett 1979).

The International Olympic Committee Medical commission was formed in 1967 and given the task of setting up an antidoping program. The commission published a list of banned compounds in time for the 1968 Olympic games in Grenoble, France, and Mexico City, Mexico. The list consisted of only four groups of drugs: psychomotor stimulants, sympathomimetic amines, miscellaneous central nervous system stimulants, and narcotic analgesics. However, the level of sophistication of the laboratories was not sufficient, and consequently few athletes using banned drugs were caught. Moreover, there were inconsistencies among the national and international sport governing bodies as to how and where testing would occur and what, if any, penalties would be enforced (Connolly 1984). The first large scale testing of athletes occurred at the 1972 Olympics in Munich, West Germany, where 2,079 samples were tested. The laboratory tested only for the three classes of stimulants and narcotics, but proved that a laboratory with properly trained personnel and equipment could correctly analyze a large number of samples over a short period of time.

Anabolic steroid abuse was also widespread in the 1960's and 1970's, however, the testing was far too costly and time consuming to be done on a large scale. In the mid-1970's, an immunoassay was developed as a screening method for anabolic steroids. With the new screening method available, the IOC added anabolic steroids to the banned list in 1975, and testing was begun at the 1976 Olympics in Montreal, Canada. Of 275 samples tested for anabolic steroids, eight positive samples were found. Athletes found ways to circumvent the tests by taking steroids that were not detected by this particular immunoassay. A new method for the detection of all anabolic steroids and testosterone was developed in the late 1970's using gas chromatography/mass spectrometry. This method was first used at the 1983 Pan American Games in Caracas, Venezuela, where seventeen athletes were disqualified for positive urine drug samples (Almond 1984). Testing of all athletes for anabolic steroids with the GC/MS system was first used in the 1984 Olympics in Los Angeles, where twelve of 1,510 total samples were found to contain anabolic steroids or testosterone (Catlin 1987).

On January 3, 1986, at its 80th Annual Convention, the National Collegiate Athletic Association (NCAA) adopted mandatory drug testing for athletes by the addition of Amendment 30 and Amendment 107 to their constitution. Amendment 30 outlines disciplinary action and testing procedures, and Amendment 107 provides for the financial cost of drug rehabilitation for athletes (Rovere 1986). A list of substance metabolites and generic equivalents was prepared (based on the IOC list), and the use of these agents is prohibited during athletic competition. The NCAA list of banned compounds now consists of six main categories: psychomotor stimulants, sympathomimetic amines, anabolic steroids, beta-blockers, diuretics, and street drugs. Many prescription and over-the-counter medications contain or are metabolized into prohibited substances, thus producing a positive result. (See Exhibit A for NCAA banned list and refer to NCAA Banned Drugs Reference List for a more comprehensive list.)

Drug Categories

Central Nervous System Stimulants

The three categories of central nervous system stimulants are the psychomotor stimulants, miscellaneous central nervous system stimulants, and the sympathomimetic amines. Methamphetamine, phenylpropanolamine, and caffeine are examples of this group. Although these drugs produce psychological and physical stimulation in athletic performance, their physiological side effects can be detrimental. They produce aggressiveness, anxiety, and tremor, which can lead to poor judgment placing the individual at risk of injury. Heart rate and blood pressure can be increased causing dehydration and decreased circulation. Complications from these side effects include the risk of cerebral hemorrhage (stroke) or cardiac arrhythmias (heart-beat irregularities) that can result in cardiac arrest and death.

Greater than 15 mcg/ml (micrograms per milliliter) of caffeine in the urine is considered illegal by the NCAA. (The USOC lowered their limit to 12 mcg/ml in February 1986.) To reach this limit one would have to consume approximately 10 cups of coffee in one sitting. Other sources of caffeine, including the following examples, are listed to indicate how excessive levels might be inadvertently accumulated:

2 cups coffee = 3–6 mcg/ml
2 colas = 1.5–3 mcg/ml
1 No-Doze = 3.6 mcg/ml
1 Aspirin, Empirin, or Anacin = 2–3 mcg/ml
1 cup Guarana tea will reach the banned level

Anabolic Steroids

Anabolic steroids are derivatives of the male hormone, testosterone. They increase protein synthesis which can, with training, create an increase in lean muscle mass. This is perceived by athletes to increase strength and endurance. Anabolic steroids, being hormones, interfere with the normal hypothalamic-pituitary-gonadal axis of hormonal balance.

This interference of normal hormonal function produces detrimental side effects.

The major side effect in the adolescent is premature closure of the growth centers. Effects in the adult male include: increase in aggressiveness and sexual appetite, sometimes resulting in aberrant sexual and criminal behavior, testicular atrophy and cessation of spermatogenesis, enlargement of the breasts, premature baldness, and premature enlargement of the prostate gland. Long-term effects include liver dysfunction, cystic degeneration of the liver, cancer of the liver, and premature hardening of the arteries and high blood pressure, which can lead to early stroke and heart attack. In the female, anabolic steroids can cause irreversible masculinization, abnormal menstrual cycles, excessive permanent hair growth on the face and body, enlargement of the clitoris, and deepening of the voice.

Executive Regulation 1-7-(b)

The following is the list of banned drugs:

I. Psychomotor and central nervous system stimulants:

amiphenazole
amphetamine
bemigride
benzphetamine
caffeine[1]
chlorphentermine
cocaine
cropropamide
crothetamide
diethylpropion
dimethylamphetamine
doxapram
ethamivan
ethylamphetamine
fencamfamine

meclofenoxate
methamphetamaine
methylphenidate
nikethamide
norpseudoephedrine
pemoline
pentetrazol
phendimetrazine
phenmetrazine
phentermine
picrotoxine
pipradol
prolintane
strychnine
AND RELATED COMPOUNDS

II. Sympathomimetic amines[2]:

clorprenaline
ephedrine
etafedrine
isoetharine
isoprenaline

methoxyphenamine
methylephedrine
phenylpropanolamine
pseudoephedrine
AND RELATED COMPOUNDS

III. Anabolic steroids:

boldenone
clostebol
dehydrochlormethyl-
  testosterone
fluoxymesterone
mesterolone
methenolone
methandienone

nandrolone
norethandrolone
oxandrolone
oxymesterone
oxymetholone
stanozolol
testosterone[3]
AND RELATED COMPOUNDS

IV. Substances banned for specific sports:
Rifle:

alcohol
atenolol
metoprolol
nadolol

pindolol
propranolol
timolol
AND RELATED COMPOUNDS

V. Diuretics:

acetazolamide
bendroflumethizide
benzthiazide
bumetanide
chlorothiazide
chlorthalidone

hydroflumethizide
methylclothiazide
metolazone
polythiazide
quinethazone
spironolactone

ethacrynic acid   triamterene
flumethiazide   trichlormethiazide
furosemide   AND RELATED COMPOUNDS
hydrochlorothiazide

VI. Street drugs:
     heroin   THC (tetrahydrocannabinol)[4]
     marijuana[4]

Definition of positive depends on the following:
1. for caffeine: if the concentration in urine exceeds 15 micrograms/ml.
2. refer to Section No. 3.5 of the Drug-testing Protocol or Executive Regulation
   1-7-(c)-(5).
3. for testosterone: if the ratio of the total concentration of testosterone to that
   of epi-testosterone in the urine
   exceeds 6.
4. for marijuana and THC: if the concentration in the urine of THC metabolite
   exceeds 25 nanograms/ml.

The most common steroids in this class are nandrolone (Decca-Durabolin), methandienone (Dianabol), stanozolol (Winstrol), oxandrolone (Anaver), and testosterone. The presence of any amount of anabolic steroid or their metabolites is illegal. Since testosterone is a naturally occurring steroid, a special condition has been placed upon it. In normal subjects the ratio of endogenous testosterone to another steroid, epi-testosterone, is approximately 1:1. An athlete with a testosterone/epi-testosterone ratio greater than 6:1 is presumed positive for testosterone.

Beta-Blockers

Beta-blockers are drugs commonly used for heart disease to lower blood pressure, decrease the heart rate, and block stimulatory responses. They are used in sports such as shooting to steady the trigger finger.

Diuretics

The misuse of diuretics in sports under certain circumstances, such as making weight in boxing or wrestling, is potentially dangerous. They may produce muscle weakness, gastric irritation, light-headedness and dizziness, muscle spasm, transient blurred vision, and headache. A common diuretic is furosemide (Lasix).

Street Drugs

Street drugs are included due to their dangerous nature and the fact that they are illegal, controlled substances. Common street drugs are methamphetamine (speed), cocaine, and marijuana.

Collection Protocol

The collection procedure used by the NCAA and the U.S. Olympic Committee was designed with strict chain-of-custody to ensure sample integrity throughout the collection and testing procedures. The sample identity is known only to the governing bodies.

The athlete is usually notified of the test immediately after competing, and is given one hour to report to the collection facility. An athlete signature form is filled out with a personal history and a declaration of all drugs taken recently (prescription or over-the-counter). This declaration is used to identify possible banned compounds before the actual testing of the sample. A collection container is randomly selected to prevent any deliberate tampering. Collection of the urine specimen takes place under the direct observation of a trained attendant. The athlete must produce a urine specimen of at least 100 mls. Sodas and water are available for those who cannot produce the required volume of urine. The athlete chooses two sample containers which will become known as the A- and B-samples. The A-sample is tested immediately, while the B-sample is frozen for later analysis in the event of a legal challenge. The urine is poured from the collection container into the two sample containers, while retaining a small amount of a pH and specific gravity test. These two tests ensure that an unadulterated specimen has been collected. Unacceptable specimens are rejected and another specimen will be collected. The samples are capped and a numerical code attached to each container. It is important that the athlete verify that all numbers on the sample containers and the paperwork match. The samples are sealed into shipping containers and sent to the laboratory for testing.

Analytical Methods

A number of analytical techniques are employed for the detection of drugs in body fluids. The most common are immunoassay, chromatography and mass spectrometry. Each technique offers distinct advantages for the detection of individual drugs or classes of drugs (Moffat, 1986).

Immunoassay

Immunoassay techniques have become a very popular method for the detection of drugs of abuse from body fluids. They are techniques that exploit the principles of immunology. There are a number of different kinds of immunoassay, including radioimmunoassay (RIA), enzyme multiplied immunoassay technique (EMIT), enzyme linked immuno suppression assay (ELISA), and fluorescence polarization immunoassay (FPIA). The immunoassay uses antibodies to locate and bind to any drug that is present in the sample. An antibody is a protein created by the immune system that has the ability to recognize a specific antigen, such as another protein, a virus, or a drug. These antibodies are commercially raised in animals, usually sheep. This is done by injecting the animals with a drug-protein complex, and separating the resulting antibodies from blood. Antibodies can be tailored to recognize broad classes of drugs, such as all barbiturates, or by very specific and detect only a single barbiturate, such as phenobarbital.

The assays use common procedures for drug detection, however, each has a different measurement technique. In the initial stages of the procedure, antibodies are mixed with a urine sample, and any drug present in the urine will form a drug-antibody complex. A tagged drug is then added to the mixture, and competition for the antibody takes place. The amount of tagged drug captured by the antibody is proportional to the amount of drug originally in the urine sample. In RIA (radioimmunoassay), the tag is a radioactively-labeled form of the drug. The amount of radioactivity remaining after further processing is a measure of drug originally present in the urine. RIA is extremely useful in dirty samples, where other constituents of the sample might interfere with the measurement. In EMIT (enzyme multiplied immunoassay technique) the label is an active enzyme. A competition between the drug in the urine sample and the added enzyme-labeled drug is established. The amount of unreacted enzyme-labeled drug is now free to further react with a third chemical resulting in a color change. This color change indicates the amount of drug present in the urine sample. FPIA (fluorescence polarization immunoassay) is similar to RIA, however, the tagged drug is labelled with a fluorescent-compound instead of with radioactivity. The amount of polarized light of a specific wavelength is measured to determine the amount of drug present.

Chromatography

Chromatography is a method of separating a complex mixture into individual components. Separation takes place in a matrix with properties for retaining the compounds of interest. The rate of movement of a compound through the matrix is unique. A mixture will separate into individual components, due to the characteristic retention properties of each component. The different types of chromatography used for the detection of drugs are: thin layer chromatography (TLC), high performance liquid chromatography (HPLC), and gas chromatography (GC).

TLC

Thin layer chromatography is the oldest of the analytical methods available for drug detection. It is a rigid plate, usually glass, covered by a thin layer of silica or alumina. A drop of sample extract is applied or spotted at one end of the plate and dried. The plate is developed by placing it into a solvent bath, with the spotted-end immersed in the solvent. As the solvent moves up the plate in a wicking action, much like a sponge absorbing water, drugs are carried along with it at different rates. The result is a separation of the sample into individual components. The drugs in the sample are detected by spraying the plates with chemicals which react with the drugs to form characteristically colored spots. The distance the spot moves from the origin is measured by a term called *RF*. Each drug will have a unique RF and color change for identification purposes. The advantages of the TLC system are that it is cheap, fast, and does not require expensive equipment. The disadvantage of this technique is its lack of sensitivity.

High Performance Liquid Chromatography

High performance liquid chromatography (HPLC) is a technique in which a solvent is forced through a column filled with a packing material. A sample is injected into the column and forced through it with the solvent. The drugs will move through the column at different rates, resulting in a separation of the mixture. The time it takes a drug to go from the front of the column to elution is known as its retention time. Each drug will have a characteristic retention time. The detection of the drug is usually accomplished by a UV-detector that senses those compounds that absorb a specific wavelength of ultraviolet light. The advantages to liquid chromatography are that the retention times of the drugs are very reproducible, and therefore offer much greater specificity than techniques like TLC. The use of the UV-detector allow quantification of the drug and also added specificity by choosing a wavelength characteristic of the drug being looked for.

Gas Chromatography

Gas chromatography is the most widely used form of chromatography for the separation and detection of drugs. A gas, usually helium or hydrogen, is the driving force which moves the molecules through the column. Each component will have a different affinity to the matrix of the column, and be retained for some unique time. The affinity of the compound to the matrix is temperature dependent. As the temperature is raised, the molecules of a particular species will become too volatile to be retained on the column and will be carried away by the gas to a detector.

The most common detectors are flame ionization detectors (FID) and nitrogen phosphorus detectors (NPD). The NPD will detect only those compounds that contain either a nitrogen or phosphorous atom and is particularly well suited for the detection of drugs of abuse, since most contain nitrogen atoms. An even more discriminating detector is the mass spectrometer. It can detect molecules by monitoring specific masses.

Mass Spectrometry

The most sensitive and specific technique for the identification of drugs is mass spectrometry (MS). A sample passes through a beam of electrons, causing the molecules to fragment into smaller pieces. These pieces are measured, and a graph of the fragment masses versus relative abundance is plotted. This graph is the mass spectrum and is a unique fingerprint for each drug. All drugs found by one of the screening methods, immunoassay or chromatography, are confirmed on the mass spectrometer for positive identification. When coupled with a gas chromatograph, the resulting technique, GC/MS, offers both the separation and retention time properties of the GC and the absolute identification of the drug by the mass spectrometer. It is virtually impossible to misidentify a drug with this amount of information, making GC/MS the most legally defensible method available.

170

Summary

Any use of drugs by athletes is prohibited by the NCAA, and immediate loss of eligibility will result if the athlete tests positive. Further, any person helping an athlete take a banned substance will be subject to equivalent penalties to the fullest extent possible.

References

Almond, E.; Cart, J.; and Harvey, R. (1984) Olympians finding the drug test a snap. *Los Angeles Times* Part III/Sunday, 29 Jan. 1984.

Beckett, A. H. and Cowan, D. A. (1979) Misuse of drugs in sport. *British Journal Sports Medicine* 12:185–194.

Catlin, D. H.; Kammerer, R. C.; Hatton, C. K.; Sekers, J. H.; and Merdink, J. L. (1984) Analytical chemistry at the games of the XXIIIrd Olympiad in Los Angeles. *Clinical Chemistry* 33(2):319.

Connolly, H. (1984) Fair play through drug test? *Muscle & Fitness* Feb. p. 90.

De Merode, A. (1979) Doping tests at the Olympic Games in 1976. *Sportsmedicine,*

Moffat, A. C. ed. (1986) *Clarke's isolation and identification of drugs.*

Percy, E. C. (1978) Ergogenic aids in athletics. *Medicine and Science in Sports* 10(4):298–303.

Rovere, G. D.; Haupt, H. A.; and Yates, C. S. (1986) Drug testing in a university athletic program: Protocol and implementation. *Physician and Sportsmedicine* 14(4):69–76.

United States Olympic Committee. (1986) *USOC/IOC banned drug list* ed. R. O. Voy, 15 Jan 1986. Committee on Substance Abuse, Research, and Education.

CHAPTER 9

SPORT PSYCHOLOGY: AN ALTERNATIVE TO DRUGS IN SPORT

David L. Cook, Ph.D.

At no other time in the history of sport has the topic of drugs been so relevant. In the recent 25th Olympics in Seoul, this fact became very evident (Johnson and Moore 1988). Our society has placed such a premium on athletic excellence that athletes are tempted to do whatever it takes to gain the winning edge. In some cases this means turning to drugs for performance enhancement. Athletes are frequently rewarded handsomely for their success despite any unethical means that they may have used. Therefore, the message these athletes receive encourages them to continue to compete in this unethical manner.

A large number of athletes view drugs as a shortcut to success or as an escape from the pressures of the game. Many of the conventional means which have been used for these reasons have been scrapped because of the time or effort required. Athletes are sold a philosophy that time is always running out, and they had better do today whatever it takes to get ahead. This attitude unfortunately de-emphasizes the immediate physical and emotional health of the athlete.

If this trend is continued, it is inevitable that sport as we have known it will cease to exist. The issues surrounding drugs in sport are critical not only to the lives and health of the athletes, but also to the life of sport. In a sense—we could "kill two birds with one stone." We must consider this possibility carefully, because the stone is in the hands of many athletes who are naive as to the consequences of their actions.

The purpose of this chapter is to explore the alternatives to the use of drugs in sport. What are the new trends in sport psychology which offer healthy and ethical solutions to the athlete's situation. Are these techniques practical, logical, and are they efficient, relative to the time constraints of the athlete. This chapter will attempt to provide viable alternatives to the serious athlete so that the athlete can say "no" to drugs because "I have a better way."

Affects and Effects

Athletes use drugs for several reasons. Many people, including some coaches, assume that athletes are no different than the normal population in their reasons for drug use. As we read in Chapter 1 of this text, athletes are a specialized population, and therefore may be at risk for reasons other than those we consider when thinking of the normal student.

There are basically two broad categories under which drug use by athletes could fall. The first category could be called the *affects* category. The reason an athlete may use drugs could be for performance enhancement—to affect performance in a positive direction. The second category could be called the *effects* category. An athlete may use a substance in an effort to help cope with the effects of the sport. Let's look at the affects category first.

Performance enhancement is a primary reason an athlete might turn to a drug supplement. Athletes are looking for ways to increase strength, recover from workouts more quickly, increase energy output, and increase endurance. These reasons for using drugs are somewhat different than those for the normal population, and should be of utmost concern to those involved in sport. Every athlete has the goal of improving in each of these areas. Improvement in one or more of these areas means a greater likelihood for success. Coaches spend much of their time trying to figure out how to get the athlete to put out the tremendous effort that it takes to improve in each of these areas. A very dangerous rationalization made by many athletes is that a pill is much easier to swallow than a tough workout, or that a hard workout followed by an injection will increase chances for success. With the pressure to improve in sport, it is not surprising that these short-cut drugs have become an option to the athlete. What is unfortunate is that this decision, in most instances, is an uninformed decision. The costs have not been identified or counted.

The second category has to do with the effects of sport on the athlete. Sport in America has become big business and big business is synonymous with high pressure. Whenever the issue of money infiltrates an activity, many of the original ideals fall by the wayside. In many instances in collegiate sport, the ideals of fair play and healthy competition have succumbed to the win-at-all-costs model. Winning, among other things, means money, and success in our society is equated with the dollar. University athletic programs cannot function without revenue. Loyalty to a school will put a few people in the stands, but winning will fill the stands. Therefore, as we whittle down this problem, we find the athlete at the center of the issue. To please the fans, to put people in the stands, to provide money for the continuation of the athletic program, the team must win. A tremendous amount of pressure is placed on the athlete to perform to the highest standard each week. Here is where the initial pressure originates.

Because the athlete is also expected to be a student and to stay eligible, a second pressure is added. Travel to and from athletic contests causes an athlete to miss a significant amount of class. The rigors of practice cause an athlete to study and function as a student in a fatigued state. Socially, the athlete is on stage at all times and must therefore, be cognizant of being a role model.

Furthermore, athletes have to constantly cope with the possibility of injury. Injured athletes have to deal with the physical pain of the injury as well as the emotional trauma of falling behind and the loneliness of rehabilitation. This becomes the third major stressor to the college athlete.

There are many more pressures which athletes must face, but these three illustrate the effects of sport on the athlete. When the pressures become too great, individuals will look for release. In the case of many athletes, the release is sought through the use of alcohol or other drugs. It is important for those involved in athletics to be aware of the origin of this negative coping behavior so they can help teach healthy alternatives.

Sport Psychology as an Alternative

The field of sport psychology has emerged in recent years because of the tremendous importance placed on the mind in performance. Many universities have faculty and courses in this area. The primary purpose of the Sport Psychologist is to provide information to coaches and athletes which will enhance their performance and help them to cope with the effects of sport. Keeping in mind that athletes turn to drugs for performance enhancement and coping, sport psychology has, as its very purpose, healthy alternatives to the issue of drugs in sport.

In the area of performance enhancement, sport psychology offers techniques and strategies which an athlete can use to increase concentration, confidence, and motivation. Strength coaches tell us that the key to success in the weight room is concentration and motivation. Athletes who do not believe this, or who lack self-discipline in these two areas, will sometimes turn to steroids as their answer to this problem.

In the area of coping with the effects of sport, sport psychology teaches effective stress management and coping skills. These skills prepare an athlete for on and off the field stress, as well as how to deal with injury rehabilitation. Sport psychology prepares the athlete for the obstacles that will be faced on and off the field. In many cases, it is these obstacles which cause an athlete to turn to an outside source such as drugs for escape, instead of looking for effective coping strategies.

Alternatives to Drugs: Performance Enhancement

In this section of the chapter, several alternatives will be discussed. It is intended that this discussion be a brief introduction to these ideas. The interested athlete may respond to these ideas by seeking further information through the university Sport Psychologist, or by checking out a text from the library on the techniques of sport psychology. It must be understood that there is no magic in the field of sport psychology. It is the dedication of the athlete to the application of the techniques, which will allow victory over the enticement of the drug world.

Positive Self-Talk

The principle of positive self-talk asserts that the most influential messages that we will ever receive come from our inner conversation, not from what others might say to us. In other words we are in a constant dialogue with ourselves, and this dialogue greatly influences our actions (Schwartz 1986). Self-confidence, which is a critical element in performance, is also based significantly on what we communicate to ourselves. Our self-talk then becomes one of the foundation blocks of success.

Many athletes may begin using performance enhancing drugs because they do not believe in their ability to perform as well without a supplement. This negative belief is conveyed over and over, until the athlete is convinced to try the drug. It is common to see this happen with the use of steroids. Typical self-talk might go something like this.

176

"I'm not gaining strength quickly enough. If I were stronger I would surely be more successful. My chances for success on the field would increase, and the coaches and scouts would think highly of my prospects. I've noticed others in the weight room gaining strength quicker than I am, and they don't seem to be putting out as much effort as I do. It seems unfair. I bet they are using steroids. All the other teams must use them too, because they all seem to be bigger and faster than I am. I bet I'm one of the few not using steroids. If I'm going to keep up, I better consider using them. Besides, I don't see others having any adverse reactions to them. Also, the coaches don't seem to care how we gain strength, just that we do. In fact, I know that some of those guys in the weight room getting the pats on the back and winning the lifting recognition awards are on the *juice.*"

The preceding self-talk is a typical inner conversation that a collegiate athlete may have many times over. If in fact we are influenced by our self-talk, then this athlete is at high risk for making the decision to use steroids. A simple technique for combatting negative self-talk is called *thought-stoppage*. Thought-stoppage teaches the athlete to become aware of self-talk, understand its power, and begin controlling it.

A simple method for teaching thought-stoppage is to fold a piece of paper into three sections. Label the first column "situation," the second column "typical response," and the third column "mental toughness response." It is important to do this in a non-emotional setting so that a clear perspective can be achieved. The idea is to think back over various competitions and recall the situations which caused a lapse in concentration, a distraction, or a self-defeating emotional reaction. These are to be listed in the first column. Next, move to the second column and briefly describe the typical negative mental response to each situation (i.e., self-talk which was being conveyed). Next, go to the third column and develop a mental toughness response to each situation.

Mental toughness can be defined as the ability to respond to adversity with positive self-talk during the heat of battle. The mental toughness response should not merely be a token positive response, but a realistic self-enhancing statement. This will keep the mind focused on thoughts which will not hinder the body from performing. Remember, thoughts control movement, and movement defines performance. Our thoughts, therefore, are the basic foundation block for performance.

Though this process seems very simplistic, it is difficult to execute in the heat of battle. Once an athlete has taken the time to go through this initial process in a non-emotional setting, the mind has a greater likelihood of responding effectively during performance. The key is to set the mind in a habit of positive self-talk. This happens by realizing typical thought patterns in specific situations and then being able to choose thoughts, instead of allowing the circumstances to dictate a negative response.

In terms of the enticement of drugs in sport, thought-stoppage can be a very effective deterrent. The athlete can recall the situations in which thoughts of using drugs were most prevalent, or anticipate situations where the pressure to use drugs will be the greatest. In either case, the process described above will allow the mind to begin developing a positive rationale for not using drugs and will strengthen the athlete's self-talk in each situation. The athlete will in fact be producing a mental toughness response to the decision of drug use. It can be seen that a strong drug education program is an important ingredient in this process, so that a strong rationalization for not using drugs can be programmed into the athlete's self-talk.

The foundation of making a change, or anticipating the need to make a stand, is having the ability to control self-talk. In fact, the key ingredient to most problems is to have the ability to cope in this manner. Therefore, dealing with the issue of drugs comes down to one basic point: does the athlete have the ability to choose to control his or her response to the situation. This can be done by choosing effective self-talk.

Goal-Setting

Another alternative to drugs in sport is developing a detailed goal-setting program which includes a drug-free plan for success both on and off the field. An athlete who has taken the time to develop a blueprint for success will be less likely to turn to a gimmick during the process. It is the athlete with little foresight who responds to the question of drug use with an emotional, rather than an intellectual, process.

Research indicates that goal-setting does in fact enhance an individual's chance for success (Locke et al. 1981). If goals are written, specific, both long-range and short-range, and are shared with others, there is a high probability that they will be reached. Because of this fact, it follows that an athlete can use goal-setting to combat the question of resorting to the use of drugs.

Goals are especially important for strength training. In the weight room goals are one of the greatest motivators. If an athlete has a daily, weekly, and monthly target to strive for, and if the athlete can see progress through conventional means, the likelihood is lowered for turning to steroids. Many athletes who resort to steroids fail to have drug-free goals, and therefore are at risk for reaching for what they consider to be a short-cut to success. An athlete who has seen goal-setting work will understand the work-effort-success connection, and will be less likely to give in to the short-cut mentality.

Goal-setting is also important to the team as a unit. It can be beneficial for a team to take a stand together on the issue of drugs by setting team goals in this area. It establishes peer pressure not to use drugs and lends itself to accountability among teammates to adhere to the goals. In an age where peer acceptance is highly valued, this can be used as an effective tool to counter the use of drugs. Not only does this process help to bond a team, but it also makes difficult choices easier to deal with by giving an athlete an immediate excuse to say "no."

Imagery

A third alternative to using drugs in sport is to explore the use of imagery for performance enhancement (Nideffer 1976). Imagery has become a popular topic in the news recently because many Olympic and professional athletes have discussed its positive effects on training and performance. Imagery is the precreation of an upcoming competition or event by using positive visualization. This process allows the athlete to establish confidence by envisioning success rather than hoping for success.

Imagery enables the athlete to experience the game many times before the actual contest. It establishes positive self-talk and provides a way for the athlete to see how strategies and goals will be accomplished. It helps the athlete feel comfortable with the environment and prepared for the particular distractors associated with the facility. Imagery allows the athlete to arrive at the game feeling like he or she has been there many times before, and that the outcome has been established. This enables the athlete to compete aggressively with confidence, rather than with doubt or fear.

The use of imagery can also significantly improve practice time. It has been said "perfect practice makes perfect." To have a perfect practice, an athlete must arrive in the right frame of mind. One way of achieving this is to take time before practice to concentrate on what is to be accomplished. The athlete can use images of intense concentration and positive work habits to prepare the mind for a positive practice and to clear the mind of distractions. Because practice to a large degree predicts performance, using imagery to prepare the mind for practice may be the most important use of this technique. Concentration and motivation are the keys to having a good workout in the weight room (Cook 1985). Imagery can be used as a method to help prepare the athlete's mind to concentrate and be motivated to work. Imagery can therefore become an alternative to steroids for the athlete who is willing to rely on inner strength rather than an injection.

There are several key elements for imagery to become a positive mental training tool. The first is that the images must be positive and realistic. Unrealistic images may not be believed by the athlete, and therefore will have little impact on the athlete's subconscious thoughts. Secondly, the images should include pictures of the athlete overcoming obstacles which will accompany competition or workouts. This anticipation and preparation rehearsal can increase the athlete's confidence and mental toughness. Remember—mental toughness is the ability to respond to adversity during the heat of battle with positive self-talk. Visualizing the overcoming of obstacles increases the likelihood that those obstacles will be overcome in reality. Thirdly, positive images must be repeated over and over. Repeated images will leave an indelible impact on the mind, and therefore will be easy to recall during the competition.

Imagery can also directly help the athlete prepare for the possibility of being confronted with drugs. The athlete can anticipate and prepare for the day he or she may be enticed to turn to drugs for performance enhancement or pleasure. A definite plan of action can be visualized and strategies developed to say "no" to drugs when they are presented.

Remember, imagery can provide the athlete with confidence when it is time to perform. There may be no greater performance for an athlete than when that person is able and prepared to say "no" to drugs. An athlete who is committed to drug-free success is the athlete who will resort to nothing less.

Alternatives to Drugs: Coping with Pressure

The pressures of being a college student are great. This fact is even more exaggerated when the student is also a collegiate athlete. A recent NCAA survey (Nov. 1988) conducted by the American Institute for Research found that football and basketball players at Division I schools spend an average of 30 hours a week on their sport during the season. This leaves little time for studying. Furthermore, studying is usually achieved in a fatigued state. Besides the obvious time pressure, pressures from the rigors of class, pressure from the coach, pressure from self-expectations, and pressure from other people's expectations can each become an overwhelming force in the life of the athlete. Athletes generally have little preparation for the challenges they face at the collegiate level. Because of this, many athletes cope ineffectively with pressure, and in many cases ruin their careers. This section will explore alternatives for coping with pressure.

The most common coping strategy for college students today is the use of alcohol (Cook and Tricker 1988). Individuals will attempt to escape from reality by drinking. They do escape temporarily, but reality is always waiting for them when they return. Many an athlete has lost a career by dealing with pressure through the use of alcohol or drugs. For some less fortunate, it was their lives that were lost.

Social Outlets

People, in general, need outlets to release stress. Athletes are no different. Positive outlets must be established which offer the athlete a positive and effective escape from the tensions which will be faced daily.

One effective outlet is that of an outside support group. Athletes should be encouraged to develop a support group of friends beyond their sport. Some coaches may view this as destructive to team unity or another distractor to athletic performance. However, having an outside support group will provide the athlete with an outlet. This outlet becomes extremely important because it functions to help the athlete keep life in perspective. John Wooden understood this concept well as he didn't believe in athletic dorms. Instead he dispersed his athletes among nonathletes. Being constantly surrounded by those who eat, drink, and sleep sport can cause the athlete to have an unbalanced sense of reality. When the only reality an individual knows is the score on the scoreboard, the pressure can become almost insurmountable.

Athletes who become single-minded to the point that "all their eggs are in one basket" frequently develop a fear of failure. This evolves because their identity becomes defined exclusively by their performance on the field. Fear of failure produces an inordinate amount of pressure. It leads an athlete into playing—not to lose—rather than playing to win. A victory merely becomes avoiding failure once again, while a loss is seen as a measure of self-worth. Athletes who perform with this attitude hanging over their heads will most likely fail to reach their potential.

There must be an outlet for these athletes, or they will continue to relate their entire self-worth to athletic performance. The outside support system discussed above is one outlet. It provides a potential opportunity for athletes to have their identity defined outside of sport, thus providing a much needed piece to the self-worth puzzle. It is important for all individuals to have more than one piece to this puzzle. Athletes are especially at risk for a lack of pieces because of the single-mindedness demanded by the sport. Deriving identity from other sources will also lower the pressure of fear or failure. This can be done through goal-setting outside of sport (i.e., academics, future employment, student activities, church or civic involvement, etc.). The coach can go a long way in fostering this process by having the athlete write down outside of sport goals along with sport goals. This allows the athlete to be constantly aware of the other aspects of life which help define him or her. When the athlete feels like a multifaceted individual, he or she is free to perform without fear of failure. The scoreboard no longer is the definition of self-worth. When an athlete performs without this fear, performance can be significantly enhanced. Concentration can be focused on the task at hand rather than on the consequences.

Time Management

Another major source of stress is a perceived lack of time. Many athletes feel that lack of time is their greatest stressor. They perceive that there is not enough time to get everything done. In this state of mind, worry frequently takes the place of action. Simple time-management skills can help the athlete see that there is time. Developing a weekly schedule is helpful in that it frees the individual's mind to concentrate totally on the task at hand. This takes the place of worrying about how everything will get done.

Scheduling has several important aspects. It allows the athlete to visually see how the puzzle can fit together. Scheduling programs the mind so that it knows what is expected. It enables the athlete to study one subject without worrying about another, because both have been accounted for in the schedule. It helps the athlete concentrate during practice, knowing that time has been scheduled for studying later. Also, athletes will find that by scheduling they will find some much needed free time. Free time is imperative for the mind. By scheduling an hour or so of free time each day, the athlete creates an opportunity for the mind to take a real break. Without scheduling, free time is spent worrying about things that have not been done, or is wasted by feeling guilty for relaxing.

Again, the concept of time-management may seem insignificant when one discusses the pressures of sport and drug use. But the fact remains that student athletes are escaping through the use of alcohol and drugs. Many of these athletes are feeling so behind in class, or overwhelmed by the amount of work to be done in a short period of time, that they look for the most convenient outlet. And many times that outlet is alcohol. If an athlete copes in this fashion, grades suffer, pressure mounts further, more ground is lost, and the athlete will likely respond by drinking more. Time-management is a tremendous safeguard against this scenario.

Recreation and Relaxation

Another fact about stress is that pent-up tension or pressure will eventually lead to debilitating problems. The final suggestion of this chapter is to develop a tension-release coping strategy. This can be achieved through any non-stressful recreational activity, such as fishing, hiking, reading, surfing, etc. Hobbies or activities similar to the ones mentioned above are healthy ways to release mental and physical tension. These types of activities provide diversions which can free the mind of stress and worry. During the week of competition, an athlete may find that a recreational diversion is not feasible because of time constraints and lack of physical energy. It is during these times that a knowledge of relaxation training techniques would be most beneficial.

There are several relaxation training strategies which teach people the skill of alleviating built-up stress (i.e., progressive relaxation, autogenic training, etc.). Each technique helps the person detect excess stress and then rid the body and mind of it. Relaxation training helps those individuals, who do not have time for another form of release, to have a readily available coping strategy. It can be very helpful for athletes to use relaxation training on and off the playing field (Nideffer 1981). On the field it helps them regulate arousal and tension. This regulation sharpens the athlete's concentration and alleviates debilitating tension. Off the field it provides healthy pressure release for the athlete in a situation where another outlet is not feasible.

Summary

Several alternatives to the use of drugs in sport have been discussed. This brief list is only a small sample of the many alternatives available. These alternatives, like the others, will equip the athlete to say, "No . . . because I have a better way." We cannot effectively legislate athletes' decisions, but we can equip the youth of America with effective coping skills and outlets when the pressures they face become unbearable.

Young athletes, therefore, should be introduced to the sport psychology skills that have been discussed in this chapter and others. These positive life skills not only can provide performance enhancement on the field, but they also can become the catalyst for saying "no" to drugs off the field. If sport is truly a training ground for life, then we should ensure that our athletes are exposed not only to physical skills training, but also to psychological skills training.

References

Cook, D. L. (1985) Motivation for resistance training. In *Muscular fitness through resistance training*. T. R. Thomas, pp. 39–42. Dubuque, Iowa: Eddie Bowers Pub.

Cook, D. L. and Tricker, R. (1988) Recreational drugs and the student athlete. *NCAA Drug Education Video Program* NCAA. Kansas City, MO.

Johnson, O. and Moore, K. (1988) The loser. *Sports Illustrated,* Oct. 88, Vol 69(15) pp. 20–27.

Locke, E. A.; Shaw, K. N.; Saari, L. M.; and Latham, G. P. (1981) Goal setting and task performance: 1969–1980. *Psychological Bulletin* 90:125–152.

Nideffer, R. M. (1976) *The inner athlete: Mind plus muscle for winning.* New York: Thomas Y. Cromwell Company.

Nideffer, R. M. (1981) *The ethics and practice of applied sport psychology* Ithaca, NY: Mouvement Publications.

Schwartz, R. M. (1986) The internal dialogue: on the asymmetry between positive and negative coping thoughts. *Cognitive Therapy and Research* 10:591–605.

Suggested Readings

Curtis, J. D. (1987) *The mindset for winning* LaCross, WI: Coulee Press.

Leohr, J. E. (1986) *Mental toughness training for sports* Lexington, MA: Stephen Greene Press.

Orlick, T. (1986) *Psyching for sport: Mental training for athletes* Champaign IL: Leisure Press.

Syer, J. and Connolly, C. (1987) *Sporting body sporting mind.* Englewood Cliffs, N.J.: Prentice-Hall.

Index